African Arguments

Written by experts with an unrivalled knowledge of the continent, African Arguments is a series of concise, engaging books that address the key issues currently facing Africa. Topical and thought-provoking, accessible but in-depth, they provide essential reading for anyone interested in getting to the heart of both why contemporary Africa is the way it is and how it is changing.

African Arguments Online

African Arguments Online is a website managed by the Royal African Society, which hosts debates on the African Arguments series and other topical issues that affect Africa: africanarguments.org

Published by Zed Books and the IAI with the support of the following organizations:

The principal aim of the **International African Institute** is to promote scholarly understanding of Africa, notably its changing societies, cultures and languages. Founded in 1926 and based in London, it supports a range of seminars and publications including the journal *Africa*.
www.internationalafricaninstitute.org

Now more than a hundred years old, the **Royal African Society** today is Britain's leading organization promoting Africa's cause. Through its journal, *African Affairs*, and by organizing meetings, discussions and other activities, the society strengthens links between Africa and Britain and encourages understanding of Africa and its relations with the rest of the world.
www.royalafricansociety.org

The **World Peace Foundation**, founded in 1910, is located at the Fletcher School, Tufts University. The Foundation's mission is to promote innovative research and teaching, believing that these are critical to the challenges of making peace around the world, and should go hand in hand with advocacy and practical engagement with the toughest issues. Its central theme is 'reinventing peace' for the twenty-first century.
www.worldpeacefoundation.org

About the author

Paul Richards is an anthropologist with over forty-five years' experience of living and working in West Africa. He is emeritus professor of technology and agrarian development at Wageningen University in the Netherlands and adjunct professor at Njala University in central Sierra Leone. His previous books include *No Peace, No War: An Anthropology of Contemporary Armed Conflicts* (2005).

EBOLA

HOW A PEOPLE'S SCIENCE
HELPED END AN EPIDEMIC

PAUL RICHARDS

ZED

Zed Books

LONDON

In association with
International African Institute
Royal African Society
World Peace Foundation

Ebola: How a People's Science Helped End an Epidemic was first published in 2016 by Zed Books Ltd, The Foundry, 17 Oval Way, London SE11 5RR, UK.

www.zedbooks.net
www.internationalafricaninstitute.org
www.royalafricansociety.org
www.worldpeacefoundation.org

Typeset in Haarlemmer by seagulls.net
Index: ed.emery@thefreeuniversity.net
Cover design: Jonathan Pelham

A catalogue record for this book is available from the British Library.

ISBN 978-1-78360-859-1 hb
ISBN 978-1-78360-858-4 pb
ISBN 978-1-78360-860-7 pdf
ISBN 978-1-78360-861-4 epub
ISBN 978-1-78360-862-1 mobi

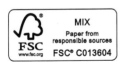

To Esther Yei Mokuwa, and all citizens of the three Ebola
epidemic countries, Guinea, Liberia and Sierra Leone, in
acknowledgement of what they endured, and what they learned.

À Esther Yei Mokuwa et à tous les citoyens des trois pays touchés
par l'épidémie d'Ebola : Guinée, Liberia et Sierra Leone, en
reconnaissance de ce qu'ils ont enduré et de ce qu'ils ont appris.

CONTENTS

FIGURES AND TABLES

Figures

Tables

ACKNOWLEDGEMENTS

Ebola Virus Disease in coastal Upper West Africa (Guinea, Liberia and Sierra Leone) in 2013/15 was an event that caused local devastation and global alarm. Some commentators predicted a pandemic with millions of cases. The rapid decline of the epidemic was perhaps as unexpected as its sudden arrival. Massive intervention by aid donors, medical volunteers and scientific researchers began during the second half of 2014, and made an invaluable contribution to the decline of the epidemic. But this part of the story is well known from media documentation. A less well-known aspect is how the epidemic played out on a local level, and in what ways local responses helped (or hindered) attempts to slow its spread. This is the theme I attempt to pursue in the present book.

I was an anthropologist in the field when the epidemic first arrived. It was an unprecedented event in the region, and my instinct was to try to document the rapid learning process required to address the challenge of the disease. This book has been written with unusual haste to capture some lessons learned. I should add that I am not a medical anthropologist, so I write primarily as an ethnographer, with some familiarity with domestic and social conditions in the countries concerned.

My debts to those who have guided or corrected my attempts where I venture on to specialist medical and epidemiological terrain are very large. In particular, I am grateful for the help provided by the reviewers of the manuscript, and by two colleagues who have been especially diligent in their efforts to ensure I passed muster in molecular matters – Daniel B. Cohen and Lina M. Moses.

Participation in the British-based online Ebola Response Anthropology Platform (www.ebola-anthropology.net) was also very helpful to my understanding of the social dimensions of the epidemic. Stephanie Kitchen of the International African Institute is thanked for her outstanding editorial support. My single biggest debt is to my life and research partner, Esther Yei Mokuwa, and her team of courageous fieldworkers: Joseph Amara, Nancy Bassie, James Bockarie, Sao Bockarie, Jestina Conteh, Sahr Fayia, Emily Gamanga, Sonny-Boy James Mokuwa, Jonathan Johnny, Francis Baigeh Johnson, Fomba Amara Kanneh, Kadiatu Kanneh, Vandi Kanneh, Wisdom Keifala, Philip M. Lahai, Christian Lansana, Sheku Moiforay, Gelejimah Alfred Mokuwa, Josephine Sannoh, Idrissa Sesay, Roland Suluku, Mamawa Tarawali and Jimmy Tengbeh. They collected much of the evidence discussed in Chapters 4 and 5, while I was out of action with complications resulting from a bad malaria attack. All those who guided and assisted me have my heartfelt thanks, but of course they must also be absolved from errors that may remain.

Why the epidemic abated as it did continues to attract debate. The international response was certainly a major contributing factor. It is possible that acquired immunities – about which we as yet know little – may have played an important part. This book argues that the local response was also significant in mitigating spread of the disease. It is essential to understand community capacities for social resistance to disease, and how better use might be made of these capacities in confronting future emergent disease threats.

Njala University, Mokonde, Kori chiefdom,
Sierra Leone, February 2016

INTRODUCTION

Ebola[1] is a disease of social intimacy. Infection spreads among those who care for the sick, including those who prepare the dead for burial. There is no cure, or treatment beyond palliative care. Death rates can be as high as nine in ten cases. Discovered in central Africa in the 1970s, the Ebola virus has caused around twenty known outbreaks to date, all in Africa. An outbreak in Upper West Africa in 2013 quickly turned into an epidemic, the world's first, mainly affecting Guinea, Liberia and Sierra Leone. This book tells the story of that epidemic, and draws lessons. Specifically, it argues that a need to understand Ebola poses a challenge for every citizen and every community at risk, and not just for medical science.

The disease

The reservoir for the Ebola virus is maintained in animal populations in the African forests, perhaps species of bats. From time to time, humans living on the margins of these forests become infected, possibly as a result of hunting animals carrying the virus. This initial crossover is known as a spillover event. Further transmission occurs when carers or sympathizers come into contact with the body fluids of someone sick with Ebola. To halt human-to-human spread patients need to be isolated and communities quarantined.

The virus is not airborne, and thus Ebola is not very contagious. It can be conveyed only by contact with the body fluids of an Ebola victim. Peter Piot, one of the discoverers of the virus, stated that he would not fear to sit next to an Ebola case on the London Tube, provided the person was not actually vomiting.[2] Unfortunately, however, Ebola is highly infectious. One droplet of body fluid absorbed through mouth, nose or eyes, or a cut in the skin, is enough to transfer the disease.

The Ebola virus was acquired by germ-warfare laboratories during the Cold War, and feature films have been made about what an escape might entail. A global panic was sparked by the arrival from West Africa of airline passengers with the disease in Europe and the United States in mid-2014. Predictions were made of millions of deaths within months. Several governments, including those of Britain and France, suspended flights from the region, and helped mount an international effort to contain the disease, undermined, of course, by the flight bans they had imposed. But whoever said government was a coherent art?

The doom-laden predictions did not come true. Liberia, the worst-affected country a year earlier, was declared free of the disease in mid-2015, though there have been three case clusters in that country since, probably related to the longer-than-anticipated survival of the virus in certain body fluids such as breast milk and semen. Guinea and Sierra Leone were declared Ebola free by the World Health Organization on 7 November and 29 December 2015 respectively, but like Liberia have seen some localized and quickly contained outbreaks linked to survivors.[3]

Effectively, the epidemic has now ended, and international attention has turned to other things. But a short memory with regard to Ebola is foolhardy. The lessons of Ebola need to be thoroughly understood, including lessons about the need for broadly based factual understanding within populations, and not just among experts, as a framework for control.

This is because Ebola attacks the very basis of family life – the daily care we provide for each other. In particular, it punishes those who care for the sick. In the complex and ceaseless web of global interactions this is a perverse sanction on those who are most assiduous in exercising their social duty. This perversity matters for us all, for mutual care fosters stable communities, and thus stable interaction between communities.

Ebola might have, but did not, destroy social cohesion in the three countries subject to the epidemic. Entire communities might have been scared into mass flight, but were not. Affected groups stood together and addressed a common threat. Local agents and international responders, working together, discovered something not known hitherto – how to end an Ebola epidemic.

The rest of the world ought to ponder the courage and commitment to community values displayed by these actors in reducing the Ebola threat. What would have happened if Ebola had coursed through neighbourhoods in London or New York? Would the local population have stood so firm? Or would social dereliction and disorder have been widespread?

More specifically – and this is key – would urban populations in the 'developed' world have formed such an effective combination with medical responders as emerged in the villages and slums of Upper West Africa? It thus seems important to ask how, precisely, that combination emerged.

A people's science

Epidemiology is a people's science. Everybody has to get involved. Below a certain threshold of participation mass vaccination campaigns cease to work. Fear that a control programme has hidden motivations or unacknowledged consequences – that polio is secret sterilization, or that the childhood 'triple' vaccination causes autism – can wreak havoc with the statistical effect necessary to halt spread of a disease.

And statistical effects are at times among the hardest concepts for humans to grasp. They often clash with what we think we know, personally and individually. It is this presumed personal knowledge that powers rumours. The consequences of Ebola are seen as evil. So it cannot be a kindly touch that spreads the disease. There must be demonic forces at work. And so we cast around and rather easily find the evidence, chosen from a large repertoire of ideas we maintain to link risk and blame.[4] Immigrants, other countries, bad leadership, germ warfare or the feckless poor spring all too readily to mind.

There was a great danger that the rumour mill would defeat all attempts to control Ebola in Upper West Africa. Social media and other gossip channels of a more traditional kind were alive with plots and conspiracies. Why did the disease affect areas known to vote for the opposition, if Ebola was not a plot to rig the next election? Why did a group of US army scientists arrive in the region to take blood samples, if it was not germ warfare? And so on, on and on.

And yet in the case study examined in Chapter 6 rumours evaporated as quickly as they came. Faced with the realities of the disease the common folk learnt to think like epidemiologists.[5] As interestingly, epidemiologist began to think like the common folk. Merged understanding was crucial to epidemic control. This book explores how and why the usual small talk was often rather rapidly abandoned, and replaced by a people's science of Ebola epidemiology.

Techniques of the body

When, in mid-2014, the threat of an Ebola epidemic in West Africa loomed, there was a clamour for advanced technological solutions, from vaccines and drugs to robot nurses. Yet the epidemic was reduced not through biomedical treatments, or machines substituting for human agency, but through better understanding of what was necessary to eliminate risks of *contagious* bodily interactions.

Some lessons were applied from earlier outbreaks. But by and large things began to change positively in Upper West Africa only when communities accepted, or improvised, changes to their own established repertoires of care.

Ebola control in Upper West Africa centred on the modification of what the great French anthropologist Marcel Mauss called 'techniques of the body'. Mauss was one of the first anthropologists to develop an interest in technology, not from a love of devices and machines, but from the perspective of skill, performance and effective use of tools. He proposed to start technology studies with the analysis of the human body.[6]

This is an interesting but unusual perspective on technology, as I know from personal experience. For a number of years I taught and researched social aspects of technology from a Maussian perspective. My line caused much head-scratching, not least among my employers, who would have preferred it if I had focused on more 'relevant' topics such as the potential of nanotechnology or reducing public resistance to genetically modified foods.

My interest in technology had instead gravitated towards foundational aspects – those that Mauss's mentor and colleague, Emile Durkheim, would have called elementary (in the sense of elemental) forms.[7] The elementary forms of technology, I argued, are most readily apparent through the study of techniques of the body.

The West African Ebola epidemic is an example of why the elementary forms of technique matter. Vaccines take time to develop, and that time period is not easily shortened. International authorities lifted normal safeguarding procedures to speed Ebola vaccine development, but trials have been made more difficult by the downturn in infections. This rapid drop in numbers of people infected was a product of the rapidity with which changes in body contact and body technique were implemented.

Control of Ebola, therefore, fits well within the tradition in technology studies initiated by Mauss, of seeking to understand tools, machines and prostheses as extensions of, and not as replacements for, human agency.[8] A central prescription of this approach is never to lose sight of the hand wielding the tool, the brain behind the hand, and the socialization behind the brain. In the case of Ebola, to understand the spread of disease we need to grasp how certain embodied skills and performances are deeply bound to social contexts. Specifically, this means paying attention to topics such as how the sick are nursed, and how the dead are buried.

The argument

This book traces the response to Ebola in 2013/15. I have been asked 'why have I written a backward-looking account of the epidemic?' Would it not be better, especially as a contribution to a series labelled *African Arguments*, to discuss what Ebola implies in terms of Africa's pathetically weak health systems? Is it not the case that Ebola shows those systems need to be vastly strengthened? And is it not a scandal that elites escape for better medical treatment to the developed world, leaving their fellow citizens to suffer unaided? This approach is to ask for a study taking the facts of the epidemic as given and focusing on equity and justice. Ebola, I suggest, teaches us something different. It warns us against wilful ignorance. People's science, I argue, is the antidote to that ignorance. It is important we understand the need for people's science.

The argument will be controversial, so it is better that I state it up front. In the circumstances in which Ebola arrived in Upper West Africa better-functioning health systems might only have made the epidemic worse. Where there is no prior familiarity with Ebola, and where it takes a laboratory reference to diagnose the virus, and thus to differentiate between several competing diagnoses with symptoms similar to Ebola, such as malaria and Lassa fever, health facilities would still have spread Ebola to medical personnel and other patients (nosocomial infection), however well equipped and staffed they might have been. Imagine the rate of spread of the disease if every rural health post in Upper West Africa had possessed a functioning ambulance for referral of cases, in circumstances where there was no experience of Ebola or knowledge of the specialized nursing techniques needed to keep carers and patients safe from cross-infection.

So Ebola is less a disease of poverty than a disease of ignorance. And that ignorance has to be addressed, since it extends to us all. In particular, there are as yet no effective 'high-tech' treatments available anywhere, irrespective of how well funded or accessible to users the health system might be.[9] Patient care, even in hospitals capable of the highest levels of biosafety standards in the developed world, requires the same kind of palliative response offered by a tent in the bush – rehydration therapy and relief of symptoms.

A further important point to be grasped is that Ebola is one of a family of emergent diseases. These are ones where humans or domestic animals become exposed to pathogens through moving into a new environment, or where the pathogen has mutated. This means that in every such outbreak responders are, to a degree, groping in the dark. Response and knowledge must co-evolve.

In the initial outbreak of Ebola in Guinea in December 2013 even the experts in emergent viral diseases were wrong-footed. For a time they placed undue stress on the risks posed by forests and hunting, with the result that many people thought themselves safe from infection because they lived nowhere near a forest, or never ate the bushmeat supplied by forest hunters.

Perhaps the key area of ignorance concerned technologies of burial. It turned out that one of the drivers of the epidemic was participation in large funerals. These were (in the terms of the responders) 'super-spreader events'. Large funerals were, in particular, a feature of the powerful male and female sodalities (so-called secret societies) widespread throughout much of the Upper West African forest belt. Yet the burial procedures for society elders were known only to society members, who were sworn to secrecy. Thus a priority for Ebola control was to enlist the support of the sodalities. Only members knew the practices and could thus properly assess and respond to the risks.

There was also a problem that external responders at times confused burial ritual with the processes of preparing the body for such rituals. In much of the region there are no professional undertakers. The family prepares a dead body for burial. It is this preparation, not the funeral itself, that poses the main infection risk when an Ebola death has occurred.

In the developed world do-it-yourself burial is confined to a long-forgotten history. Few, even among the anthropologists, ever sat down to make systematic accounts of body-handling techniques involved in burial practices. Funeral rites are covered in the field notes of anthropologists because ritual is a focal concern; but the practices of undertaking are often a blank page.

And yet it turned out that body-handling was one of the key infection pathways powering the Ebola epidemic. It also turned out that this was everyday knowledge among the communities. Responders had but to ask. Once anthropologists did ask – once popular knowledge was shared – it became much clearer what needed to be done to end transmission.

Attention will also be given in this book to what the anthropologist Mark Hobart has termed the 'growth of ignorance'.[10] By this, he means the wilful cultivation of this condition as an aspect of human development. We generate ignorance when we choose not to know.

A British politician once stated that the taxpayer could no longer afford to fund irrelevant anthropological studies of prenuptial practices in the Upper Volta.[11] Ironically, it has now cost the British taxpayer dear to understand the perhaps equally esoteric-seeming topic of the post-mortem practices of communities in regions neighbouring that great West African river.

A specific instance of the cultivation of ignorance, relevant to the Ebola epidemic, concerned home nursing. To international responders this topic was taboo, since it would encourage people to care for their loved ones at home instead of having them transferred to a biosecure care facility.

Nevertheless, the likelihood of home nursing was clear. The disease has two phases – a 'dry' and a 'wet' phase, both of which last for about three days, until death or onset of recovery. Patients are relatively safe to be moved during the dry phase, but Ebola is not yet apparent because the symptoms are hardly different from those of malaria. Any movement in the 'wet' phase would be highly hazardous, unless undertaken by a specialized team with protective gear and an Ebola ambulance. Few patients would seek help from a treatment centre until the diagnosis was obvious. But the only patients who could be reached were those living in areas with cell phone coverage (to phone a special ambulance helpline) and roads for the ambulance to travel upon.

Yet requests for a home care protocol to reduce the risks to those forced into caring for their family members *in situ* at first fell on deaf ears. I was told by one medical charity that it would be 'unethical' to produce such a protocol. It was (literally) unthinkable. However, knowledge emerged from community improvisers. One Liberian nurse, unable to find any hospital to admit her family, made protective suits from plastic sheets and bin bags, and safely nursed her father and two other family members through the crisis (see pp. 122–3).

International responders learnt from these kinds of activities, and home safety protocols were later devised (see Chapter 5). So ignorance is a choice. We choose to ignore the topic of techniques of the body at our collective peril.

Who am I writing for?

Who is the intended audience for this book? Top of my list I would place those who consider themselves citizens of the world, with an interest in the health of their global neighbours, and who, in a spirit of international solidarity, know that an epidemic disease in Upper West Africa potentially affects the health of all. Ebola is a fearsome disease, but learning how West Africans have coped with it is an antidote to fear and confusion.

Students of technology, public health and nursing are also, for obvious reasons, close to the top of my list. The book's argument focuses on embodied skill, and how new techniques of the body can be developed, in even the most challenging of conditions. All three professions just mentioned require an understanding of the nature of skill, and in particular how to change skill sets that become counterproductive. Yet too often the topic of embodied technique, and how to foster it, is downgraded relative to theoretical knowledge.

The sociologist of technique Tim Dant carried out an innovative study of British car repair.[12] He found the technical manuals remained pristine in the boss's office. Bad roads, and bad drivers, knock vehicles out of shape. Much car repair concerns the knocking of car bodies back into shape. This is not an exact science. Apprentices have to learn how hard to hit. A guiding hand is of more use than a car-repair manual.

Learning how to cope with Ebola is not an exact science either. The science of Ebola is largely a matter of having insight into the embodied experience of care, and knowing how to guide that embodiment into new, safer pathways.

In addressing skill formation and the materiality of care considerable emphasis will be placed on the need to assess social context. Every day we are bombarded with news about innovations that will – it is alleged – revolutionize our lives. Human problems will not be solved with machines alone. Ebola is a stark illustration of this message. Hands, brains, task groups and social values continue to matter as much as tools and equipment, and no study of technical (or medical) innovation makes proper sense without consideration of body technique in its social context. If Ebola epidemiology is not an exact science, it is not exclusively a medical science either; it is a social science as well.

I hope also that what I write will hold some interest for the large number of volunteers who took part in the Ebola response. I admire without reservation those who dropped everything, and were willing to risk their lives, in responding to a desperate and perplexing social need. This includes national health professionals and community volunteers from the three most affected countries, as well as the large numbers of international responders, including military personnel. What they achieved in such a short time, and against such heavy odds, in helping to create a people's science of Ebola control, is remarkable. Skilled inventiveness was an important aspect of their contribution, and this book endeavours to capture that point.

Possibly I will also retain some readers from my earlier academic work on techniques of agrarian food security, explored in the book *Indigenous Agricultural Revolution*.[13] I had originally wanted to call that book *People's Science*, until my publisher stepped in, arguing booksellers would never know where to shelve it. Fortunately, booksellers today are electronic, and have the power of modern search engines at their disposal. So now I have a second chance.

But the perspective has changed. *Indigenous Agricultural Revolution* argued that African farmers often knew more about their own environments than the scientists attempting to help them. Ebola offers a new challenge. In dealing with an emergent disease, and the world's first epidemic, neither responders nor communities knew at the outset what would work. But by collaborating to beat back the infection they generated novel shared knowledge. It is the importance of this co-production of epidemiological knowledge to which the present book draws attention.

What this book does, and does not, argue

In the following pages some evidence is provided that a downturn in Ebola was under way in some parts of the Upper West African region before the international response was fully elaborated. One reader of an earlier draft of the manuscript wondered whether I was implying that the international response was unnecessary. There are two points I need to make to guard against any such interpretation.

The first is to caution that we do not yet properly understand why Ebola faded out in Upper West Africa. There is some (as yet unpublished) evidence that some groups of people (notably family carers) may have developed a degree of immunity to the virus, and this might have helped to end local outbreaks.[14] Only with published confirmation that such immunities exist, and more detailed analysis of the local distribution and downturn in cases, will it be possible fully to assess how much of epidemic decline was driven by conscious human adaptation to Ebola infection risks. But the claim made here is that local learning played some significant part.

The second point concerns people's science. I use this label to refer to emergent knowledge concerning adaptation to Ebola risks distributed across a population comprising affected communities and local and international medical responders. In other words, to the extent that the downturn in the epidemic depended, at least in part, on conscious human adaptation, I understand it to have been a joint effect.

Perhaps excusably, in a short book, I have given some prominence to the community aspect, but only because this is the least-documented aspect of this distributed response. Equally, I make clear that community learning was at its most rapid where there were open channels of communication between communities and medical responders. Future response to Ebola and other emergent zoonotic disease challenges should pay close attention to the need for effective multilateral learning.

Chapter 1

THE WORLD'S FIRST EBOLA EPIDEMIC

Ebola Virus Disease is a severe haemorrhagic fever caused by the crossover to humans of four species of filoviruses circulating in animal vectors in African forests and forest margins. Death rates range from 25 to 90 per cent.

In December 2013 the most deadly (Zaire) species of the virus caused human deaths in the forested part of south-eastern Guinea, and infection spread rapidly to two neighbouring countries, Liberia and Sierra Leone. In twenty or so previous African outbreaks Ebola had been localized and rapidly contained. In Upper West Africa the disease spread over a much larger area and travelled (in a few cases) between continents, thus becoming the world's first Ebola epidemic.

The incubation period of the virus in humans ranges from two to twenty-one days. The course of the disease itself runs for about six days before organ collapse and death, or the onset of recovery.

The main symptoms of a first, dry phase (lasting about three days) include headache, fever and extreme tiredness, symptoms easily confused with those of malaria. In the second, wet phase the symptoms include vomiting, diarrhoea and bleeding from mouth, eyes and other orifices. No evidence has been found of airborne infection. Known infection pathways all involve direct contact with the body fluids of an Ebola patient. The virus enters through body orifices such as eyes and mouth, or through breaks in the skin.

Many dictionaries treat infection and contagion as more or less synonymous, but for Ebola a distinction can be drawn between the two terms. Ebola is highly infectious, in that the smallest droplet of blood, faeces or vomit is dangerous, as are sperm and breast milk after recovery, but the disease is not very contagious. The virus is fragile when exposed, and is not spread by casual contact. Infection occurs only in the wet stage, especially among those involved in nursing a victim or in disposing of a body.

Epidemiologists talk in terms of a reproduction number (R_n). This is the average number of subsequent infections per case. For an Ebola outbreak this number is not very high (typically about 2 – less than measles, for example). But those intimate with an Ebola patient are at high risk, since contact with body fluid is potentially lethal.

The crisis of the disease is the wet stage, a time of high risk for all attempting to care for the patient. Rehydration is important for successful patient care, but even a simple act such as refilling a drinking cup can infect the carer. Response agencies learnt to treat Ebola like cholera, also a disease with no antidote, where dehydration is a killer, and drips essential. But attaching a drip to a sick, fearful, restless Ebola patient is an extremely risky task for a nurse.

Cumbersome protective clothing is necessary (personal protective equipment, PPE). This inhibits movement, and limits the time a nurse or doctor can work in tropical heat. Learning how to put on and take off protective clothing safely is a crucial technique in Ebola epidemics. A tedious, inescapable routine must be followed to the letter, however pressing the demand. The protective dress terrified many patients, and fed rumours of germ warfare and body snatchers.

How bodies are handled in sickness and death is thus a central issue for treating Ebola patients and ending infection chains. Control calls for the rapid modification of techniques of the body on the part of all – whether lay or professional – who attempt to care for patients or handle dead bodies. In this lies the central theme of this book – how responders, and especially families and communities, acquired these modified techniques of the body.

Prior experience of Ebola

What was the state of knowledge about the disease when the Upper West African epidemic began?

Ebola first became known to science in the 1970s as the result of an outbreak in an isolated area adjacent to the Ebola river in the Democratic Republic of Congo (then known as Zaire). Early cases were associated with hunters, bushmeat and dead forest animals. Outbreaks were sometimes magnified by hospital infections.

An excellent general account of these earlier experiences is to be found in a book by two medical anthropologists, Barry and Bonny Hewlett.[1] The Hewletts studied Ebola episodes in Uganda (2000) and Congo (2003) through first-hand ethnographic field research, and collated information on all other outbreaks up to 2007. Table 1.1 summarizes this information, supplemented by data on more recent episodes from World Health Organization (WHO) sources.

The single largest episode occurred in northern Uganda in 2000 (425 cases). Other outbreaks were mainly small, and confined to isolated forest or forest-edge communities. Infection pathways were often traced through hunters coming into contact with infected (sometimes dead) animals, such as chimpanzees and duikers. Fruit bats were identified as symptomless carriers of the virus.

The Uganda episode stands out not only as the largest outbreak in numbers of persons infected (prior to 2013), but also in being urban based. Previous episodes had been in remote, rural localities. The Gulu outbreak made clear some of the new challenges associated with outbreaks in more densely settled communities.

The response to the epidemic of 2013/15 had to face the challenge of how to respond to Ebola in both isolated rural conditions and also in densely crowded urban areas. There were large numbers of cases of Ebola in the capital cities of Guinea, Liberia and Sierra

Table 1.1 Pre-2013 African outbreaks of Ebola virus disease (excluding single cases)

	year, cases, species	year, cases, species	year, cases, species	year, cases, species	year, cases, species	year, cases, species	Notes
DR Congo (Zaire)	1976, 318, Zaire	1995, 315, Zaire	1999, 73, Zaire	2007, 264, Zaire	2008, 32, Zaire	2012, 57, Bundibugyo	2012 not in Hewlett & Hewlett
Congo	2001-2, 59, Zaire	2002, 13, ?	2003, 143, Zaire	2003, 35, Zaire	2005, 12, Zaire		2002 not in WHO
Gabon	1994, 52, Zaire	1996, 37, Zaire	1996, 61, Zaire	2001-2, 65, Zaire			
Sudan	1976, 284, Sudan	1979, 34, Sudan	2005, 17, Sudan				
Uganda	2000, 425, Sudan	2007, 149, Bundibugyo	2012, 24, Sudan	2012, 7, Sudan			
Angola	2005, 351, ?						2005 not in WHO

Sources: Hewlett and Hewlett (2008), Figure 1.2, p. 5; WHO: www.who.int/mediacentre/factsheets/Fs103_ebola; elsewhere Angola outbreak reported as Marburg virus disease, Andrew Meldrum, *The Guardian*, 5 April 2005.

Leone. Each of these metropolitan regions contains populations in excess of one million. The spread of Ebola in urban slums such as the West Point district in Monrovia posed unprecedented challenges.

The issue of how Ebola jumped the rural–urban divide is raised in the book by the Hewletts. They discuss a theory, widely believed locally, that the infection spread into Gulu town from Ugandan army personnel fighting Hutu rebels in DR Congo, perhaps through the repatriation of the body of a dead soldier. This seems unlikely, since the Gulu outbreak was caused by the Sudan not the Zaire species of the Ebola virus. Even so, we do now know from Upper West Africa that long-distance movements by members of highly mobile occupational groups can cause the disease to move in rapid jumps from village to city and back again.[2]

Framing a response: social theory

The Hewletts also raise an important conceptual issue central to the question of how communities adapt to the threat of Ebola. This is the issue of how beliefs and ideas relate to action.

As we will see below, international responders in 2013–15, led by the WHO, emphasized the importance of correcting wrong information. It was assumed that if communities had correct information on Ebola risks then appropriate actions would follow. This is a contentious assumption, because it takes sides in one of the most fundamental debates in social science – whether beliefs cause action, or actions cause belief.

The debate is perhaps best known through reactions to the early work of the German social philosopher Max Weber, who proposed that modern capitalism was significantly shaped by Calvinistic religious belief. The British economic historian R. H. Tawney tackled the same topic and period of history but arrived at a different conclusion, namely that ideas and economic practices co-evolved, with (in the last instance) material factors shaping the beliefs (including religious beliefs) of early capitalists.[3]

This has set the terms for a debate between materialists and idealists ever since. Social scientists of a materialist orientation sometimes build on the work of another German social philosopher, Karl Marx. Materialists who reject Marxist historical determinism prefer a variant of materialist thinking proposed by a third great nineteenth-century social philosopher, Emile Durkheim.[4]

Durkheim argued that belief is significantly shaped by social action. What we do, and how we do it as a group, including ritual action, shapes what we think we know about the world.

A choice made between these three perspectives significantly modifies how Ebola responders approach the key topic of rapid change of beliefs and practices regarding the sick and dead.

Broadly speaking, the Hewletts follow a Weberian route. They proffer the notion of 'cultural models' or 'cultural scenarios' to explain community Ebola response. These scenarios shape behaviour. The analysis is subtle. The Acholi people with whom the Hewletts worked in Uganda have a range of available mental templates, we are told, to explain disease and to guide response. They possess a specific cultural scenario for infectious disease, which includes notions of quarantine, and this was the one they applied to Ebola, thus allowing the Hewletts to explain how community action contributed to Ebola decline.

What is not explained is how the cultural scenarios came into existence, or why there should be (in the Acholi instance) three such scenarios, not two, or seven. With no theory of how the scenarios arise it is hard to see what responders would need to do to induce a helpful response were suitable cultural templates to be lacking.

Followers of Marx, we might suppose, would focus directly on the material factors shaping an Ebola epidemic. It is this kind of explanation that is engaged when attention is directed to the low level of investment in medical services in Upper West Africa as a driver of the disease.[5]

Marxist materialist explanation is challenged when the phenomenon of nosocomial infection is taken into consideration. This is the word applied to sicknesses that arise within medical treatment environments, and at times promoted by the treatment itself. Treatment of Ebola within a hospital environment is very risky both for other patients and for medical personnel. Having a better-funded treatment environment is not the answer. Treatment has to be specifically redesigned to separate Ebola patients and to protect responders at the earliest stage possible. This requires patients and responders to share ideas and beliefs appropriate to the kinds of behaviours that minimize infection risk. How this alignment of ideas, belief and behaviour is to be attained is a key issue for Ebola response.

In this book it will be suggested that it is insufficient to pump knowledge into the heads of affected populations, in the hope that this altered knowledge will guide behaviour change. The Durkheimian tradition in social theory argues that the relationship between mental and behavioural states is complex, and dependent not (alone) on individual cognition, but also on patterns of group action and interaction.

The compulsion to care for a sick person, or to take part in burying such a person after death, depends on drivers of group activity. One of the most fundamental drivers of behavioural commitment is the collective emotional state triggered and shaped by a ritual performance.

In effect, the Durkheimian position predicts that it will not be possible to prevent risky behaviour such as participation in burial services by outlining the medical risks. This type of action will change, in terms of its epidemiological effects, only when risky practices are replaced by ritually and emotionally meaningful equivalent safer practices. Devising these safer practices is work for community groups, not radio propagandists. A communication approach will make better sense when it reports the results of successful local ritual innovation. Support is needed, in the first instance, for affected community groups to devise their own new patterns of group interaction.

Thus what I seek to do in what follows (especially in Chapters 4 to 6) is to apply a Durkheimian perspective to the issue of local responses to Ebola. Beneficial change in community interaction dynamics around Ebola did in fact occur, but in a patchy manner. Local reorganizational efforts at times lacked the well-targeted external support that might have accelerated them and made their benefits more generally accessible. It will be argued that what external responders lacked most was a clear theory of local ritual interaction dynamics,[6] and a support plan to enable communities to redirect their interaction dynamics in ways that would have been conducive to the rapid realignment of local beliefs and understandings with biosafety outcomes.

Ebola in Upper West Africa

The first recorded Ebola case in Upper West Africa occurred when a small boy fell sick and died in the village of Meliandou near the town of Guekedou (Gegedu), in the south-eastern part of the Republic of Guinea, during December 2013. The disease spread to members of the boy's family and then to medical personnel, unaware that they were treating Ebola cases. The outbreak site was not in as isolated a region as in earlier outbreaks. Ebola cases soon began to spread down busy trading routes to Liberia and Sierra Leone as well.

The cumulative incidence of cases at 8 June 2015, when the epidemic was coming to an end, is shown in Table 1.2.

These figures reveal some variation between the three countries.

Judged in terms of numbers of fatalities Liberia was the worst-affected country. The figures need to be read with some caution,

Table 1.2 Ebola cases in West Africa, 2013–15

Country	Cases	Confirmed	% cases	Deaths	% total cases
Guinea	3,669	3,237	88.2	2,435	66.4
Liberia	10,666	3,151	29.5	4,806	45.1
Sierra Leone	12,884	8,630	66.9	3,913	30.4
TOTAL	27,219			11,154	41.0
Nigeria	20	19		8	
Senegal	1	1		0	
Mali	8	7		6	
TOTAL	29	27		14	

Source: CDC, 8 June 2015. Confirmed means laboratory tested. NB transmission was still active in Guinea and Sierra Leone on 8 June 2015, but had ended in other countries listed.

however. Table 1.2 shows a higher number of deaths for Liberia than confirmed cases. The rise of cases in Liberia was especially rapid, and for a time overwhelmed treatment and testing facilities. Clearly, data-gathering was a casualty, and we may never know, very exactly, what happened in Liberia in the earlier stages of the epidemic.

Sierra Leone recorded the largest number of total cases, but had the lowest death rate, well below the 50–90 per cent mortality widely cited for infection with the Zaire species of Ebola virus based on earlier epidemics. The 'up to 90 per cent' fatality figure was widely publicized by international media in the early days of the epidemic. It seems possible that this may have deterred some sick people from seeking help, particularly before local community care centres (CCCs) were introduced and family members could keep a daily eye on the fate of their loved ones.[7]

The epidemic began in Guinea, but took longest to control in this country (transmission ended in late November 2015). Several explanations have been offered for this persistence, including deep ethnic and political tensions between government and the people of the forest zone where the epidemic began.

These tensions may have fostered scepticism about the purpose of government-backed control measures. A second factor to be considered in the case of Guinea, however, is that here there were fewer cases, assessed against a total population of 12 million, relative to Liberia, 4.3 million, and Sierra Leone, 6 million. Experience of Ebola, and the learning that goes with it, was thus less intense in Guinea. In effect, virus transmission may have endured because it continued to find populations unfamiliar with the disease and measures needed to combat it.

The epidemic in Upper West Africa undoubtedly also had a head start because the initial response, both nationally and internationally, was slow. Although unexpected, the Guinea outbreak, once identified, was treated according to protocols applied in earlier isolated outbreaks. It was assumed the same procedures would work as well with the Guinea outbreak. Insufficient attention was paid to the intensive cross-border networking that catapulted the disease in the direction of adjacent, crowded, capital cities on the coast.

Established procedures worked well when outbreak areas were themselves highly isolated. No such distance barriers applied in the Upper West African cases. The forest region was within hours of the three large coastal cities by road, and international air travel connections rapidly took the virus farther.

This speed of spread caught Ebola experts by surprise. For instance, in Sierra Leone the first cases were confirmed in late May 2014, but by July there were cases in Freetown, the capital. An epidemic in city environments, with crowded slums, was uncharted terrain, and a degree of panic ensued.

Fortunately, this concern was misplaced. A study of Monrovia suggests that there is a statistically significant tendency for Ebola cases in the poorest urban districts to lead to more infective contacts than cases in wealthier neighbourhoods.[8] But the difference is not very large, and urban slums did not prove to be the massive multipliers for an Ebola epidemic feared by some.[9]

A sense of panic overtaking the international community in mid-2014 was doubtless enhanced by widespread myths concerning the disease. Ebola has a certain sinister repute among those who model 'doomwatch' scenarios, not to mention those who watch Hollywood films.[10]

Both superpowers during the Cold War considered Ebola to be a potential biological weapon, and acquired genetic materials, perhaps mainly to try to figure out an antidote. The US Centers for Disease Control subsequently filed patents for some of the viral material it held, for vaccine development purposes.[11]

What was not known was whether Ebola would be a very good weapon of mass destruction. A virulent virus might all too readily backfire, and consume those who released it. Subsequent assessments suggested that the threat of Ebola would be more effective as a way of inducing panic than as a biological 'bomb'.

This indeed proved to be true. The threat of 'weaponized Ebola', in the public mind, undoubtedly complicated response to the West African epidemic. In May 2015 a rumour circulated that two patients in a hospital in Mosul, Iraq had contracted Ebola.[12] The fact that there was no known capacity in Iraq to test for Ebola did not dampen ensuing panic that Islamist rebels might be configuring a biological weapon.

So Guinea, Liberia and Sierra Leone found themselves fighting a war on two fronts. The first was against the first-ever epidemic of Ebola Virus Disease, but the second was a worldwide outbreak of media-inflamed Ebola Panic Disease.

A report by the World Health Organization, 'Barriers to rapid containment of the Ebola outbreak' (11 August 2014), cited fear as a major obstacle to rapid containment. The report noted that fear caused quarantined persons to flee, villagers to attack international responders, airlines to refuse to transport personal protective equipment, and courier services to refuse to transport properly and securely packaged patient samples to a WHO-approved laboratory.[13]

The British government, apparently mindful of possible adverse newspaper headlines as an election approached, halted direct flights to Sierra Leone and Liberia, against the advice of one of its own parliamentary committees.

The French government did something even stranger. Air France flights to Freetown and Monrovia were ended on account of Ebola risk, but not to Conakry. President Hollande explained it was a gesture of support for a francophone country. True, the spread of the virus in Guinea was never quite as rampant as in Liberia and Sierra Leone, but surely no one could have thought Ebola was less virulent on account of its linguistic orientation.

The three worst-affected countries, and their international partners, had to mobilize against the epidemic against this background noise.

A key step forward in the international response was when WHO declared Ebola in West Africa a Public Health Emergency of International Concern (PHEIC) on 8 August 2014. An international surge of response was then mobilized, even though it took several months before it was fully delivered.

A specialist UN agency, UNMEER, was founded to mobilize and coordinate this international response, and based in Ghana, a country without Ebola cases, but a choice perhaps dictated by the above-mentioned flight bans. French and Russian teams arrived to assist Guinea. British, Ugandan and other teams deployed to Sierra Leone. President Obama launched a major American initiative in Liberia, based around a large military mission.

Since Liberia was experiencing the most rapid rise in cases, the militarized American response began in August 2014. By contrast the surge in Sierra Leone did not fully get under way until December, when cases in that country peaked at 500+ a week, many of them in Freetown and its peri-urban fringe.

By early 2015 a trend towards decline, first apparent in Liberia in October 2014, was clear in all three countries. The extent to which this resulted from the international response, implementation of government controls, such as quarantine, local learning or epidemic 'burn-out', perhaps involving emergent natural immunities, will be discussed further in Chapters 2 and 3. Assigning probabilities to these different factors is worth attempting in order to consolidate understanding of prevention strategies relevant to any further emergence of Ebola on an epidemic scale.

Infection pathways

How did Ebola travel? Ebola has three main infection pathways. The first is termed zoonotic spillover. This pathway runs from forest animal host to human, often through consumption of 'bushmeat' (the name in West African English dialects for any kind of 'game'). Monkeys and chimpanzees can become infected with Ebola, but develop symptoms and die. Some species of bats show evidence of carrying the virus but are apparently symptom free.

Bats are sometimes eaten extensively in, for example, parts of Ghana, Nigeria and Cameroon.[14] Bat consumption is less common in and around the Upper West African forests.[15] So the apparent spillover event in the Guinean epidemic remains puzzling. It seems unlikely a toddler (the index case) would have been a bat eater. It has been suggested he might have been playing in a bat-infected hollow tree, and became infected through bat droppings, but other stories circulate locally about possible earlier infections.[16]

On the other hand it soon became clear from work on genetic mutation rates of the virus in samples collected from patients in Sierra Leone that zoonotic spillover was not giving rise to new infections.[17] The data from the mutational 'clock' were consistent with the interpretation that all further infection had been human-to-human.

Virologists traced three distinct lineages of the Makona variant of the Ebola virus in Sierra Leone, based on blood samples from patients with confirmed cases. The third lineage (SL3) emerged in mid-June 2014, and a recent study found that 97 per cent of its samples carried this variant of the genome.[18] These results 'link all Sierra Leonean ... cases to the initial introduction of [the virus] into Sierra Leone, and ... provide further evidence that all ... cases during this outbreak arose from human-to-human transmission rather than from further zoonotic introductions from an unknown ... reservoir [of the virus]'.[19] Furthermore (the same report adds), the genetic similarity of these viruses 'suggests that importation from other countries was minimal', though the authors do not rule this out entirely.[20]

The other two major pathways for infection involve human-to-human contact.

One is nosocomial (infection as a result of treatment in a hospital or clinic). Any medical facility not up to the highest level of biosecurity standards can cross-infect other patients with Ebola. This biosecurity capacity is found in only a very few hospitals in the Western world, so it should not be assumed, as some appear to have done, that nosocomial transmission makes Ebola a 'disease of poverty', spreading in run-down medical facilities starved of staff and funds. Ordinary hygiene cannot protect against Ebola. Specific practices must be implemented, based on a thorough understanding of infection risk.

The second 'person-to-person' infection pathway is through family care. Ebola is a 'nasty disease'[21] because it punishes carers for not abandoning their loved ones. The main risks, from virus load in body fluids, are encountered in the 'wet' phase of the sickness, and in preparing the corpse for burial. Without behaviour modification a patient will infect household carers, and the group involved in washing the dead body. Touching the body to say farewell, or handing over grave cloth as a keepsake, may further increase the numbers of post-mortem infections.

Some large-scale funerals of prominent persons led to the infection of scores of mourners. The initial fourteen confirmed cases in Sierra Leone, for instance, were all epidemiologically linked to the funeral of a traditional healer.[22] Agencies involved in the Ebola response in Sierra Leone later 'claimed that 70 per cent of new infections stemmed from funeral rituals'.[23]

Requirements for ending an Ebola epidemic

Six things must be in place to halt spread of infection.

1. Ebola victims must be identified (through reporting cases to a special telephone helpline, and rapid diagnostic testing).

2. Ebola-positive cases must then be isolated, preferably in a purpose-built treatment facility, with safe drainage and waste disposal; carers must have disposable protective gear (PPE), and stringent hygiene must be followed.

3. Patients need to be transported in special ambulances by trained teams, using PPE, to reduce risks of cross-infection.

4. There is a need to consider quarantine. Quarantine is controversial, but is still probably a necessary step. Households from which Ebola patients have been extracted were in many cases quarantined for 21 days and supplied with basic provisions. This sometimes proved counter-productive, in encouraging people to abscond. Local efforts at quarantine may be more relevant to disease control, being focused on the need to restrict movement into communities of strangers with unknown health status.

5. All close contacts of the sick person need to be traced and visited every day for twenty-one days to check for signs of sickness. This is a huge logistic undertaking. In Sierra Leone, for example, as of 9 June 2015, a total of 96,768 contacts had been followed up daily, each for twenty-one days (2,033 contacts did not finish the twenty-one days owing to death or other factors).

6. All deaths must be reported and 'safe burial' procedures applied. A trained team arrives to prepare the body, and wraps it in two body bags, before the funeral takes place. Swabs are taken to establish whether the death was an Ebola case. The family is allowed to witness from a distance, but the interment itself is carried out by the team. It should perhaps be emphasized that this applies to all deaths, whether from Ebola or not. All bereaved families are affected by Ebola, and not only those in which a death from Ebola has occurred.

All six areas just mentioned pose severe challenges of social acceptance. This is where the issues of social theory outlined above become relevant. The predominant approach in the response to the Upper West African Ebola epidemic in 2013/15 was to assume that ideas drive behaviour. To change ideas it was assumed that better information was required. Social mobilization was taken to mean a focus on messages.

Some commentators canvassed alternatives based on a materialist approach. According to this viewpoint the spread of Ebola was related to the inadequacy of medical provision. Better provision would have reduced the risks of an epidemic. But faced with the challenge of rapidly rising numbers of victims this was a counsel of perfection.

It might be better to approach Ebola prevention through an analysis of how collective action (including ritual action) supports belief. In particular, it seems important to analyse collective action in terms of body technique. How exactly was patient care delivered, and how exactly were bodies buried? This in turn might offer some insight into community capacity for changing relevant areas of embodied performance. The states of belief sustained by modes of collective action were in a sense of little account. What mattered was the extent to which communities at risk of Ebola were capable of recognizing the risks posed by their existing embodied practices and to elaborate safer techniques. Messaging was less important than scope for practice.

The following chapters thus focus on two central concerns: the way in which existing embodied techniques influence biosafety in regard to Ebola infection pathways, and the scope for endogenous change in such techniques. The case is made for a people's science of Ebola control generated through rapid group learning concerning behavioural modification. Consolidating such newly acquired capacities in communities exposed to Ebola, so that they remain available over the longer term, and disseminating these skills more widely to communities not yet affected, is a suggested prerequisite for post-Ebola preparedness throughout Africa.

Chapter 2

THE EPIDEMIC'S RISE AND DECLINE

The countries most affected by the 2013/15 Upper West African Ebola epidemic – Guinea, Liberia and Sierra Leone – occupy the bend in the Atlantic coastline, and straddle the transition from forest to savanna. They share much in terms of history and culture as frontier regions of the ancient Mali empire.

There are also significant differences. These stem in particular from the distinct modern political heritages of the three countries. Guinea was a French colony, and today uses French as its language of administration. Liberia was settled by the American Colonization Society as a home for free slaves, and became an independent nation from the mid-nineteenth century. Sierra Leone was a British colony and protectorate. The colony was founded at the end of the eighteenth century as a home for free blacks who had fought with the British army in the American Revolution. The protectorate was annexed at the end of the nineteenth century.

These similarities and differences are important in understanding the spread of Ebola and the international response.

Ebola began on the forest edge, in Guinea. This area of the Upper Guinean forest was settled at an early date by Kissi and Gola people, perhaps before or consequent upon the rise of the medieval Mali empire. The ethnonym 'Gola' is said to derive from the word for a nut with stimulant properties grown on the forest edge (kola), and traded widely throughout West Africa.

Paul Lovejoy states that this is 'either an amazing coincidence or an indication that these people were identified through their participation in the [inter-regional] kola trade'.[1] The neighbouring Kissi people were also brokers in trade between forest and savanna, especially in importing cattle from the savanna.

The long-established involvement of these forest-edge people in long-distance trade makes it apparent that the Ebola outbreak took place in an area in Upper West Africa quite different from the isolated hunting regions in the central African forests where earlier outbreaks had been experienced. Local populations on the Upper West African forest edge have over time developed extensive connections through trading partnerships and marriage that have spread over considerable distances.

Three braids of trade routes carried much of this forest-edge commerce both into the Niger basin to the north and down towards the coast. One braid (linking Sierra Leone and Guinea) followed the rivers north of Sierra Leone into the interior hills of Guinea, and towards the Upper Niger. The two others ran either side of the Gola forest as far as the segment of the forest–savanna transition zone from which the recent Ebola epidemic radiated. The initial spread of the virus was down the two routes skirting the east and west of the Gola forest, branching towards the coastal capitals Monrovia and Freetown.

Family, commercial and military alliances linked communities up and down these various forest–savanna routes, and help explain some of the networking among rural communities that accelerated the spread of the virus. Clan names, marriage alliances, the regional sodalities (Poro for men and Sande for women, sometimes called 'secret societies', because their activities, including burials, are known only to members), and shared institutional laws of hospitality connecting trading partners (landlord–stranger relationships) are commonly encountered. Disparate languages and lack of centralized state authority notwithstanding, the locality from which Ebola emerged is, historically, part of a culturally and economically integrated region only latterly divided up by colonially imposed international boundaries.

The three modern states began to take shape from the end of the eighteenth century. Portuguese established the first coastal trading links with the Sierra Leone peninsula in the sixteenth century. At the end of the eighteenth century British anti-slavery philanthropists founded a refuge for British army veterans of African origin in Sierra Leone. This became a Crown Colony (in 1807) and its port city – Freetown – a major base for British anti-slave trade patrols.

Anglo-French rivalry in the hinterlands of Freetown in the late nineteenth century led to the imposition of British and French colonial administration over the hinterland of these two port cities, and the emergence of French and English as national languages in two embryonic modern states, Guinea and Sierra Leone.

Meanwhile, Liberia emerged from the linking together of a number of coastal settlements for emancipated African-Americans, founded along somewhat similar lines to the British colony at Freetown. The British settlers were never free of colonial rule. In the Liberian case, however, the repatriated slaves formed their own independent government from 1847, though not without considerable tutelage, finance and military assistance from the United States of America.

The independent Liberian government exercised little control over districts in the interior beyond a forty-mile-wide coastal belt during the nineteenth century.[2] At the end of that century both Britain and France began to entertain designs on the heavily forested Liberian interior. To protect its agreed boundaries the Liberian Frontier Force, with American military assistance, 'pacified' interior districts by force. This alienated many local communities, hitherto living independently, and triggered hostile attitudes towards Monrovia that linger to this day.

The international border between the three countries was finally settled by exchange of territory (a portion of the Gola forest) between Britain and Liberia in 1911. The old trade routes were then reshaped into today's regional transport system, with major links homing in on Conakry, Freetown and Monrovia.

Ebola moved down these three distinct systems of communication much as raw materials (minerals and forest products) drained down them in the colonial period. This tree-like communications structure is most clearly recognized in Liberia, where people have a saying that 'if we see you going we will see you come'. There are few if any lateral connections linking other centres in the country without the traveller passing through Monrovia.

Monrovia's dominance over the lives of Liberians was reflected in the way Ebola so rapidly became an urban outbreak focused on the teeming capital.

For a time, Liberia outdid the other two countries in the rate of increase in Ebola infections. If this was due to the rapid arrival of the virus in a crowded, fast-moving urban setting, then we might see the early downturn in infection, beginning first in the heavily forested interior, as reflecting the power of indigenous institutions (notably Poro and Sande) in the Liberian interior. Some evidence (to be discussed in Chapter 6) suggests that local institutions were likewise effective in enhancing capacity to manage Ebola risks in Sierra Leone.

Guinea was different. The French ruled their colonial empire in Africa directly. They created a system that based its legitimacy on French legal codes and institutions. Institutions such as Poro and Sande were not recognized by the state as part of a system of 'indirect rule', as was practised in Liberia and Sierra Leone.[3]

At independence in 1958, the Guinean leader, Sékou Touré, refused President de Gaulle's scheme of affiliation of former colonies with France. The Guinean president turned to the Soviet Union for help, and shifted the country towards a form of centralized, planned economy.

The Marxist regime waged war on obscurantism (traditional beliefs and institutions). This bore down especially hard on the people of the forest region who had resisted the spread of Islam, and retained beliefs associated with sodality membership, and respect for forest and ancestral spirits. In Sierra Leone the ruling political classes share an interior, forest background, but in Guinea the ways of thinking of the forest perhaps seem more remote to capital city elites, and long-Islamized mercantile communities.

Some of this suspicion between forest and coast was redoubled in Guinea by (the at times enforced) involvement of some forest communities in support for dissident military groups associated with competing factions in the civil wars in Liberia and Sierra Leone in the 1990s. Guinea also had its own forest-based rebel movement seeking to challenge the rule of President Lansana Conté. Conté had responded by sending helicopter gunships against the rebels.

This fraught history of relations between Conkary and the Guinean forest communities is reflected in episodes of hostility of villagers to Ebola responders, especially a widely reported incident on 16 September 2014 at Womeh, in Nzerekore prefecture, when a mixed delegation of medical personnel and government officials attempting to disinfect communities and explain Ebola risks were set upon by a hostile crowd. Eight of the responders were captured and killed.[4]

To summarize, there is a lot shared at the cultural level between communities across all three countries, but important differences are to be found in terms of national systems of governance (with Guinea remaining somewhat more closed and top-down in its systems of administration) and in patterns of integration between countryside and capital. In Guinea, Ebola was for a time enclaved within the forest region, remote in both terms of distance and mentality from the capital. In Liberia the virus very rapidly reached the capital, where downturn was assisted by a massive American military-led response. Downturn of Ebola in the interior of Liberia and Sierra Leone depended significantly on initiatives taken by strong local leaders (as will be discussed more fully in Chapter 6), especially those influential within the sodalities, where burial practices for important elders spread the disease.

Drivers of the epidemic

The Ebola epidemic in Upper West Africa began in December 2013 in the farming village of Meliandou, close to the city of Gueckedou (Gegedu), in south-eastern Guinea.[5] It took some time to ascertain that this was an outbreak of Ebola, a disease hitherto unknown in Upper West Africa. Once the virus was identified responders assumed the disease would follow a similar path to previous outbreaks in isolated forest communities in the central African forests.

In these earlier outbreaks communities had been readily quarantined, in part through their own isolation, and infection contained. A major worry was recurrent spillover of the virus from intermediate hosts such as forest primates and human populations, especially hunters. Messages about Ebola hazards were strongly focused on the risk to forest-edge communities, especially from eating bushmeat.

Surprisingly for a disease thought to be a spillover from a forest animal host to humans (a zoonosis), the districts least affected by infection, once the epidemic began to spread, were those closest to the forest. In hindsight, this can be seen as a warning that this epidemic was different. Two of the seven chiefdoms containing the Sierra Leone portion of the Gola forest, Nomo and Tunkia, had no Ebola cases. In Liberia, Gparbolu County, an administrative district containing much of the Liberian portion of the Gola forest, was also free of cases (see Figure 2.2 below).

A problem with the international Ebola response still gathering momentum at this stage was that too much emphasis was placed on reducing the risks of zoonotic spillover. Populations in all three countries were repeatedly 'messaged' about the dangers of bushmeat, to the point where this was the single most widely known (supposed) fact about the epidemic.[6] At times, people claimed they were immune to infection because, for reasons of religion or taste, they never ate bushmeat. Others were openly sceptical about the message, asking, 'if the virus was so dangerous why didn't all the animals die?'[7]

Emphasis on zoonotic risks in the early stages of the epidemic reflected a misreading of the environment where the first cases occurred. Meliandou is a farming village with a hunting tradition. Hunting is one of the markers of social identity in a country where forest communities have a history of troubled relations with savanna-based ruling elites. But the village is located on the margins of a small city (Gueckedou) where people are highly engaged in commerce, and cross the international borders with Sierra Leone and Liberia at will. Ebola in Upper West Africa first spread among farmers oriented towards trade and not towards forest subsistence.[8]

A historical vignette will help set the social scene in the epicentre of the disease. My colleague, the late Dr Malcolm Jusu, once told me that his grandfather, a Kissi warrior from Sandeyalu, in Kissi Kama chiefdom, in Sierra Leone, but adjacent to the Guinea and Liberia borders, maintained three homes, and depending on which government – French, British or Liberian – approached him for tax would relocate himself, his followers and his animals in one or other of the neighbouring countries to avoid payment.

This kind of long-established portable cross-border identity laid the basis for family networking intensified by armed conflict in all three countries in the 1990s. War either side of the new millennium visited the Sierra Leonean, Guinean and Liberian parts of the forest belt at different times. These disturbance were accompanied by much temporary shifting across borders, to seek refuge with in-laws, until peace and stability returned from c. 2005.[9]

As already noted, market-based mobility across borders is no new thing in the region where Ebola first took off. In 1893, on the eve of colonial conquest, Thomas Alldridge, a British travelling commissioner, introduced his account of what he termed an 'ordinary native market' in Kissi country, with the remark that

'I think I shall be able to show that these [Kissi] people are not at all in the wretched condition often pictured by the European imagination'.[10]

He then lists the diversity of products available for sale, bought and sold in a local currency, Kissi pennies, made by local blacksmiths. This was the first point in his journey north at which Alldridge saw ordinary periodic markets. Further south, all the trade was in the grip of colonial traders based on the coast.

Intense, locally managed forest-edge trading activity not only survived colonial conquest, but was in fact further stimulated by the exigencies of the new international boundaries trisecting the region. In 1932 the British in Sierra Leone allowed a large international market to open at Koindu,[11] at the northern tip of Kailahun District, practically on the Guinea border. This market became famous for, among other things, its international trade in African cloth. Some of this came from as far afield as western Nigeria, contributing the word *hoku lapa* ('Yoruba [woven] cloth') to the Mende lingua franca of the forest margins.[12]

Koindu market was closed because of the civil war in Sierra Leone (1991–2002),[13] and kept inactive owing to subsequent armed disturbances in Guinea (1999–2000), and in Liberia (c. 2002–04), but was revived in 2008, after the region returned to peace. A contractor funded by the European Union began building a motor road from Kenema to the district headquarters (Kailahun) 2012.[14] The road is supposed eventually to reach Koindu. To reach Koindu from Kailahun today requires a further 30 kilometres or so of travel over a single-track dirt road, alternately rocky and muddy. The at times nearly impassable state of this road contributed more than a little to the slow pace of the Ebola response.

Koindu is, then, no more than a mile or two from the two villages through which Ebola entered Sierra Leone, and these are a mere stone's throw from the international borders with Guinea and Liberia.[15] The market was once more closed in 2014, this time in response to Sierra Leone government restrictions on trade and movement.

The first officially recognized case of Ebola in Sierra Leone (25 May 2014) involved a nurse-midwife based in Koindu, who is said to have 'treated a patient from Guinea, not knowing this patient had Ebola'.[16] The closeness of Koindu to the Meliandou outbreak ought, perhaps, to have sparked an alert. Unfortunately the first message about Ebola to be circulated among chiefs in Kailahun District (in March 2014) was a warning about bushmeat,[17] not about the dangers of human cross-border contact.

Spread of cases: a brief timeline

The WHO was first notified of an Ebola outbreak in Guinea on 25 March 2014, when numbers of cases were still small. The rate in Guinea levelled off from June to August, before rising more sharply in September, and finally reaching a plateau (with a much lower level of total cases than in Liberia or Sierra Leone) in December 2014 (Figure 2.1).

Cases in Liberia and Sierra Leone were first recorded in April and May 2014 respectively, and rose sharply from August 2014, sparking international concern and a major response. In Liberia numbers began to level off from October 2014. The same bend in the curve did not take place in Sierra Leone until January 2015. However, numbers were dropping sharply in eastern Sierra Leone from as early as October 2014. This is important to note because a downturn was evident before the main (British-supported) international Ebola 'surge' arrived.

Transmission ceased in Liberia from April 2015. Sierra Leone began a countdown to the end of the epidemic in late September 2015. Guinea began its final countdown in November 2015. Momentum in Guinea was assisted by successful ring-vaccination trials of an experimental Ebola vaccine reported to have good efficacy.[18]

Figure 2.1 *Total reported suspected, probable and confirmed cases in Guinea, Liberia and Sierra Leone provided in WHO situation reports,*[19] *25 March 2014 to 3 June 2015*

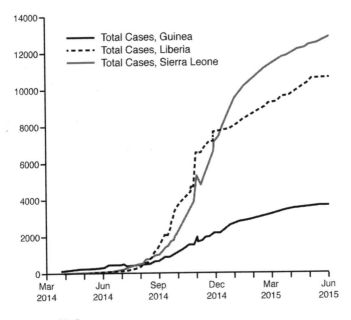

Source: CDC

Gender and age: as factors in infection

Much of the infection risk from Ebola is borne by family carers. Babes-in-arms are at high risk when the mother becomes infected. Older children are at much lower risk. WHO data show that the age group 15–44 is three to four times more likely than children to be infected, and that the age group 45+ is four to five times more likely to be infected. Not coincidentally, these are the age groups most involved in nursing the sick and processing the corpse for burial.

The gender risks of Ebola have proved harder to pin down. Hewlett and Hewlett[20] reported that females accounted for about 60 per cent of cases, based on data from earlier outbreaks. Data on adverse impacts of Ebola on survivors and survivor households for Sierra Leone[21] also show a gender split in adverse impacts. This study sampled quarantined homes (including survivors and survivor households), and found that pre-existing gender biases against women were intensified among Ebola survivors.

Age bias was also intensified. For example, there was less water-carrying by women and more by girls in quarantined homes.

But WHO data, based on records for Ebola patients in hospitals and Ebola Treatment Units, show a 50:50 split between male and female Ebola victims. This seems consistent with evidence discussed in Chapter 5 on gender responsibilities, and thus distribution of infection risks by gender, in burial. Men prepare men's bodies, and women prepare women's bodies. There is an exception; in some Muslim households washing of corpses for burial – probably the most risky task associated with funerals – is reported as a special responsibility of women, irrespective of the gender of the deceased.

In sum, it seems clear the domestic burdens of women are intensified when the woman is a survivor, or living in a quarantined household. But it is not so clear that women are more at risk of catching Ebola than men, once age is taken into account. Men and women in middle age have responsibilities to the sick and dead that put both groups at risk of Ebola infection.

Picturing the epidemic as a breaking wave

In the earliest phase (December 2013 to July 2014) the Ebola epidemic was mainly confined to places on the flank of the Gola forest (Kailahun in Sierra Leone and Lofa County in Liberia). It was soon apparent, however, that the disease was mainly spreading along main roads and through market centres, and not along the forest margins.

Ebola rather rapidly gathered impetus to reach Monrovia, Conakry and Freetown, and Ebola responders faced for the first time the prospect of a large-scale urban epidemic. This caused major international alarm. Urban slums might prove massive multipliers for the disease. In the event, these concerns seem to have been somewhat misplaced. Responding was in some ways easier in urban environments since so much in Ebola prevention hinges on logistics (the rapid putting in place of effective communications, safe transportation and safe holding centres and treatment facilities).

All three cities possess sizeable port facilities and international airports, capable of handling the influx of materials, equipment and supplies needed for Ebola Treatment Centres. Urban cell phone coverage is good, and many city roads have been improved since the end of the Mano river conflicts of the 1990s. Urban community structures proved to be not noticeably less effective than their rural counterparts in supporting activities requiring citizen support, such as case-finding and quarantine.[22]

In all three countries, however, political responses were marred by delay. Fear of being blamed for the epidemic seems to have affected judgements. For example, the president of Sierra Leone did not visit Kailahun District, the disease epicentre in that country until 28 and 29 July 2014, six weeks after the outbreak was first reported, owing apparently to concerns that it was a heartland of the main political opposition.

Likewise, the government of Liberia appeared initially to have decided that the West Point slum in Monrovia was a no-go area, and ringed it with troops, who opened fire on protesters challenging quarantine. Later it became apparent that West Point had its own community structures, and that these were already effectively engaged in the fight against Ebola.[23]

Matters were perhaps most complicated in Guinea, on account of the long-term stand-off between central government and forest communities. Local suspicions of the political motives of central government in declaring an Ebola emergency clearly prolonged some infection chains in the Guinean forest zone.

Some differences in epidemic trajectory can be noted as a result of these variations in local political response. In Sierra Leone there was a prolonged period of rural spread with an eastern focus. Government agencies talked of trying to make Kenema a barrier to spread in the rest of the country, much as there was talk in 1991 of trying to stem a feared rebel advance by dividing the country along a line separating north and south.

But the barrier was all too readily breached by high-risk contacts, reacting against chaotic conditions for Ebola patients in the Kenema government hospital. Again, in recapitulation of the tactical circumstances in the civil war, fixed army checkpoints along the main road proved no deterrent to bike taxi riders prepared to explore bush path diversion, when paid well enough by quarantine 'jumpers'.

In Liberia there was little the authorities could do to hold the epidemic wave at bay. The disease was a massive problem in the capital almost as soon as it had taken off in the interior.

Safe burial proved an immense challenge to the authorities in Liberia, who opted for a highly unpopular policy of compulsory cremations. Even so, 'safe burial' protocols were easier to implement when the bulk of cases were in one place. There were 2,000 Ebola cases in Liberia in August 2014. In the same period Sierra Leone had only 900 cases, but many of these were in rural areas inaccessible at the height of the rains. Kenema had, at the time, only one ambulance for 'safe burial', and it took up to four or five days to respond to some cases in villages. Faced with such delays, villagers took matters into their own hands, with unauthorized burials triggering further cases of infection.

Even allowing for these nuances, however, the overall advance and decline of the epidemic is surprisingly similar across all three countries. The pattern can be likened to a wave – building, breaking and then ebbing. Infection ebbed first in places where the wave had gathered. Evidence of this is contained in three maps, Figures 2.2–2.4.

Figure 2.2 Where Ebola has been

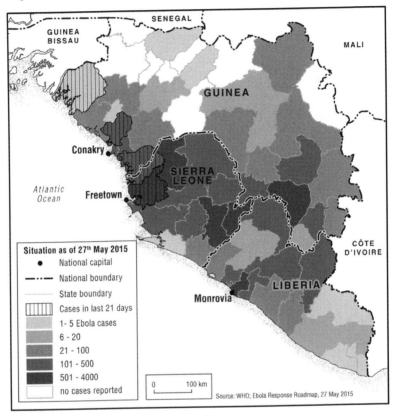

Figure 2.2 shows all localities where Ebola was or had been present up to May 2015; the disease reached almost all areas of all three countries apart from highland Guinea. Figure 2.3 shows the epidemic at its peak in late September 2014, with transmission still taking place in early-infected districts and also beginning to lap against some of the outer districts. Figure 2.4 evidences a general retreat of the disease in all early infected districts (including the whole of Liberia) by May 2015, with an active 'edge' of advance remaining across north-western Sierra Leone and coastal districts of Guinea, and reaching as far as the borders of Guinea-Bissau in the north-west.

Figure 2.3 Situation at 25 September 2014

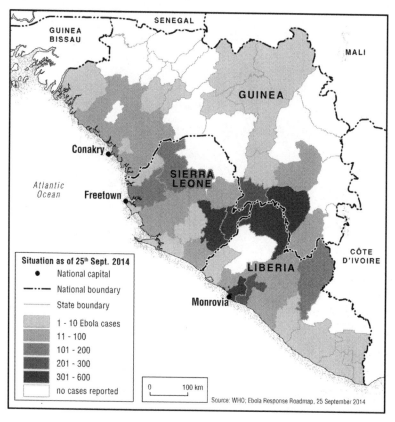

If localized variations in ecological, ethnic or political factors had driven the epidemic it seems unlikely they would have generated such a consistent wave-like pattern of early onset and early decline consistent across countries that are in many respects as different as they are similar. Seemingly the maps imply something common to the disease itself, such as burn-out due to a build-up of natural immunity, or a shared aspect of human response.

Acquired immunity among household carers has been reported, but the data have not yet been published.[24] The linearity in the maps might also be explained in terms of logistics; clearly, responders built up their assets most rapidly in districts where the disease was

Figure 2.4 Situation at 27 May 2015

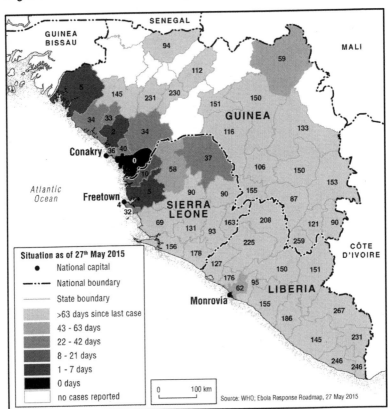

most apparent. But there is also evidence (examined in Chapter 6 especially) that local response played a part in shaping the pattern of advance and retreat. Here the argument would be that communities figured out most rapidly how the disease worked, and what they needed to do about it, in places where caseloads were highest, and (in some cases) where access to external help was limited or delayed.

Of the residual factors, probably most attention should be paid to road transportation. The data for Sierra Leone are especially informative. Figure 2.5 maps the epidemic in Sierra Leone as it was in November 2014. Figure 2.6 shows the country's main road system. The disease appears to have made a grand circular tour, starting in

Figure 2.5 Extent of Sierra Leone epidemic in November 2014

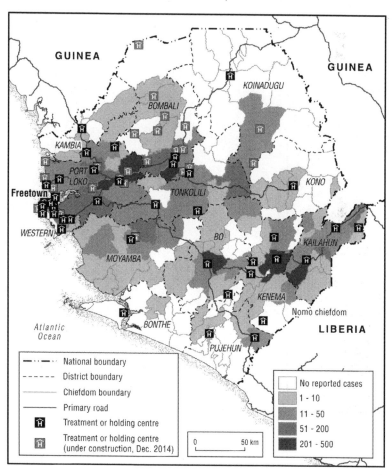

Kailahun, reaching Freetown and then spreading back up the main road system to the north of the country, finally completing the tour by arriving in the diamond districts bordering Kailahun on the west.

Clearly, properties of the transportation network were an important factor in the spread of Ebola at the national level in Sierra Leone. Areas on dead-end branches of the national road network seem to have been best able to keep the disease at bay. Pujehun, Bonthe and Koindaugu districts only ever recorded handfuls of cases.

Figure 2.6 National road system, Sierra Leone

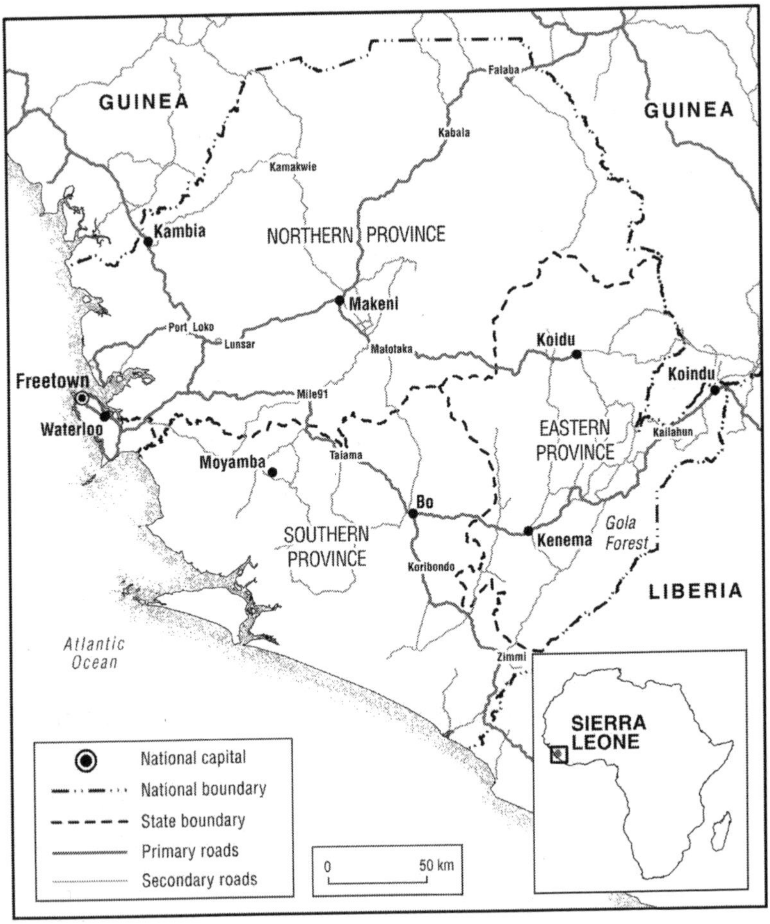

Why social knowledge is important

Models are powerful tools in capturing the relevant features of an epidemic and provide projections to guide the planning of an epidemic response. But a model is only as good as the assumptions that go into it.

On 26 September 2014 the US Centers for Disease Control predicted that there might be up to 1.4 million Ebola cases in Liberia and Sierra Leone by 20 January 2015.[25] The figure includes a correction for assumed under-reporting. There is also an important caveat that the number applies only if there are no additional interventions or changes in behaviour. Thus the prediction should perhaps be best understood as a warning rather than a projection.

The actual numbers of cases, in late January 2015, were as follows: Liberia, 8,524, and Sierra Leone, 10,491.[26] In short, the model results were wildly wrong. But the caveat shows us what we should look for if we want to know why – namely, we need to consider the additional interventions and changes in behaviour that ended the epidemic. This is the theme for the remainder of this book. But to approach that theme it is helpful to explore in what respects the model was wrong. What becomes clear is that the model failed to incorporate relevant social information, including the extent to which carers acquired immunity.

Ebola is not airborne, but is spread only by contact with body fluids from a patient in the last phase of the disease. The risks of infection are largely confined to those nursing an Ebola sufferer, or involved in handling the body immediately after death. As noted above, such risks are mainly borne by older members of the family. Even neighbours are relatively safe, provided they keep a distance. In other words, risk of infection is not randomly distributed across the population, as the model assumes, but is strongly clustered. The risk is in fact largely confined to the immediate social group intimate with the Ebola patient. Models adjusted for social assumptions about the social clustering of infection risks yielded much lower predictions of epidemic growth.[27]

However, it is important also to point out that social intimacy does not always equate with residential proximity. Many families in Upper West Africa have rural origins, but live across a rural–urban divide. Ebola is, for this reason, capable of making unexpected jumps – unexpected, that is, to those unfamiliar with the geographical ramifications of the rural African extended family.

Research has documented these ramifications with regard to an apparently isolated outbreak in the remote village of Fogbo in Kori chiefdom, central Sierra Leone, in August 2014.[28] Fogbo is situated on the Teye river, about eight kilometres by bush track from the main road running across central Sierra Leone from Freetown to Kenema. The first case in Fogbo was that of a man infected in Kenema, who had sought treatment from a member of his family in Fogbo, about 150 kilometres to the west. The man's relative was a renowned herbalist.

There is no road to Fogbo, but the village can be accessed by motorcycle taxi along tracks leading to the far side of the river, crossed by canoe. Experiencing malaria-like symptoms, the sick man feared cross-infection with Ebola if he was hospitalized in Kenema. Evading checkpoints, he travelled to the village of his family member to receive local anti-malaria treatment. In Fogbo it is apparent that he succumbed to Ebola.

The man's sickness triggered a local outbreak. The herbalist caring for him developed Ebola, and the family rallied to help her, but she died. Traders participating in the subsequent funeral of the herbalist took the disease back to the main road at Moyamba Junction, a main node for business in the area. A dispenser who had treated several of the Fogbo cases without realizing the risk then caught the disease, which was catapulted as far as Freetown when members of the dispenser's Masonic lodge came to participate in his funeral. Ebola had reached from Kenema to Freetown in two bounds in a matter of days.

Long-distance movement in Upper West Africa was until recently restricted to motorable roads. But in recent years even off-road villages have been reached by motorcycle taxis. These bike taxis were a new phenomenon in Sierra Leone and Liberia after the civil war. Many of the bike riders were self-demobilized ex-combatants, unafraid to penetrate deep into the interior.[29] There are today few villages in the three countries without some kind of motorized bike access.

The implication of the case material just discussed is that patterns of family interaction, and knowledge of how social knowledge is drawn upon to regulate these interactions, are highly relevant to any understanding of how Ebola moves. Modelling for Ebola needs to take account not only of clustering of risks due to family intimacy but also the jumps stemming from the enhanced mobility of members of the extended family group.

This poses an immediate problem for Ebola control. How can the disease be kept within localized pockets, without further pockets being cloned wherever high-risk contacts have intimate social connections.

One factor supporting Ebola control was already in place, throughout the three Ebola-affected countries. Rural people know those living around them very well, and this social knowledge serves to identify many of those who pose infection risks. A long-established institution of 'landlord' and 'stranger', widespread across the region, whereby any visitor comes under the protection of a member of the community, serves to keep family heads and chiefs apprised of movements of visitors into a settlement.

In all parts of rural Sierra Leone, for example, the presence of a stranger has to be reported to the chief, before that person is allowed to reside in a community, even for a night. This is to ensure the stranger is not maltreated, and that the stranger does not maltreat others. The requirement to report to the chief applies to persons arriving in a community to seek treatment for a medical condition.

A recent history of civil war across the region boosted this long-established rural system of social scrutiny. Villagers were alert to guard against infiltration by rebel spies and advance guards. Ebola has strengthened the legitimacy of this traditional monitoring system.

Urban and peri-urban communities also tend to reproduce the familiar village landlord–stranger system where they can. But landlord–stranger ties are less thoroughly applied in urban settings.

In villages, strangers are readily noticed, and the eagle eye of the chief will soon be drawn to an unreported lodger. Visitors in an urban or peri-urban setting are much more numerous, and much more anonymous. Even so, neighbours are less anonymous than in large cities in Europe or America, and as a result Ebola contact tracing proved surprisingly effective even in urban areas.

Major exceptions are the mining camps and roadside trading centres, where people often come and go at will. Even so, chiefs will still often attempt to supervise visitors in these places because they have a financial incentive to do so. This is especially true in alluvial mining settlements in Sierra Leone or Liberia, where the chief belongs to a landowning family. The landowners participate in a share of the finds, and keep a close eye on those who might have diamonds or gold in their pocket. I knew one chief in Tongo Field, a long-established diamond area in Kenema District, who built his house with verandas at both back and front, in order better to scrutinize the adjacent workings without leaving his chair(s).

However, it is apparent from the Fogbo case that the landlord–stranger system is no guard against the spread of Ebola through family networking. As knowledge of Ebola risks intensified during the course of the epidemic, family movements often became subject to greater scrutiny, but the claims of family often overtook Ebola fears. Even in the countdown to the end of the epidemic some high-risk contacts were still evading contact tracing procedures, presumably accommodated by family members, perhaps unaware of their high-risk contact status. So any model for Ebola needs to spread the clustering of risks around family members, but also allow for some unexpected jumps consistent with the complex networking of Upper West African family life.

In short, to understand the dynamics of the Ebola epidemic in Upper West Africa it is necessary to understand the local social response. Analysis of this response is the task attempted in the remaining chapters.

Chapter 3

WASHING THE DEAD: DOES CULTURE SPREAD EBOLA?

Few were quite as blunt as the Australian minister for immigration and border protection, Peter Dutton, who justified an entry ban imposed on visitors to his country from Upper West Africa on the grounds that 'West African ... funeral rites make those travellers an unacceptable risk'.[1] But he was not alone in implying that local cultural practices had turned an outbreak into an epidemic. A Ugandan doctor evacuated from Sierra Leone to Germany with Ebola, and a survivor of the disease, commented that 'many locals seem unwilling to break with age-old customs such as communal dining [eating from a single plate] ... [As infection mounts] people learn lessons. Unfortunately that takes a long time.'[2]

It was widely presumed that Ebola was spread because people in Guinea, Liberia and Sierra Leone stubbornly adhered to dangerous traditional beliefs. This led the international Ebola response to seek help from anthropologists, presumed to be experts in understanding culture, and thus (it was also presumed) well placed to help persuade people to abandon harmful 'age-old customs'. Maybe, for example, anthropologists could help stop people washing dead bodies, or collectively eating rice from a single plate?

But this was to put the problem the wrong way round. People do not bury bodies because they want funerals. They want funerals because they have a dead body. Washing a corpse in an Ebola epidemic is a very dangerous practice. But it also turns out that epidemiologically safe burial is unsafe from a social and spiritual perspective. An unwashed body thrown in the ground in a body bag[3] is likely to leave in its wake a great deal of social disquiet. The issue is both to prevent the washing, and to address the social disquiet.

The first part seems easy. The government of Sierra Leone made the washing of corpses a criminal offence, punishable by two years in jail. Liberia imposed cremation. But draconian approaches only added to social disquiet. Perhaps unsurprisingly, it was after the law against washing bodies was passed that response agencies began to refer to 'hidden bodies' and 'secret funerals'. People were taking the law into their own hands. Death laid upon them a higher moral imperative. The problem, as the anthropologists tried to convey, was that staying safe in an Ebola epidemic cannot be attained without also addressing the social challenges of death. As will be shown, gaining recognition for this point of view was hard. A key conceptual difficulty had to be overcome concerning what, exactly, we mean by words like culture, tradition and belief.

Is culture a cause (of anything)?

There are many definitions of culture, but by and large anthropologists use the word to refer to shared values, patterns of behaviour and material artefacts, transmitted through learning, and deployed in social interaction. The notion of a culture is a useful descriptive device.

However, it is problematic to imply that a group of people is the outcome of its culture. It is certainly true that anthropologists, at times, tend to imply that cultures are causal in more than just a metaphorical sense, as when, for example, they speak of 'acculturation'. This usage implies that an individual cannot perform as a member of a group until a common set of rules has been internalized. But in such cases it might be better to speak of acquiring a culture much as one acquires a language. I speak English, but it is not the case that

English causes me to speak. The culture is the product of people acting as a group, and not the other way round.[4]

The distinguished anthropologist Clifford Geertz did more than most to promote 'culture' as a quasi-causal variable useful in organizing large bodies of descriptive anthropological data (something he referred to as 'thick description'). For Geertz, there was (for example) no such thing as universal common sense. Common senses vary from society to society, since contexts differ, so Geertz[5] finds it convenient to bring common sense under the rubric of culture. What he seeks to say by this move is that much of what passes for 'common sense' is not universally shared but applies only within a specific setting. Polar bears are dangerous animals, but it makes little sense to be scared of polar bears in a tropical forest.

When the Hewletts wrote their pioneering book on the anthropology of Ebola outbreaks, they wanted to find a way of making their account as accessible as possible to undergraduate students of medical anthropology. So they made use of the concept of culture, which was a word familiar even to beginner students of the subject. But they were aware of the trap of assuming that culture was equivalent to 'tradition', and determined a 'fixed' response to the disease. In fact, their evidence was that when people in east and central Africa were first threatened by this new and unprecedented danger, they were highly flexible in the way they went about selecting explanations.

So the Hewletts preferred not to talk about culture as such but about 'cultural scenarios'. In the case of the Ebola outbreak at Gulu in northern Uganda, they discovered that the Acholi people had three basic models of disease, and applied them according to the nature of the evidence. Two of these scenarios relate to Acholi beliefs in spirit forces; a third approximates to epidemiological understanding. But as noted above, there was no clear explanation of what causes the epidemiological model to be chosen, except by some process of elimination. Apparently, the Acholi have a preferred order of application, because it was only when the first two models failed to explain the facts of the Ebola outbreak that the Acholi turned towards the epidemiological explanation.

Elsewhere the Hewletts use the notion of cultural scenarios both to explain why some people resist Ebola safety controls, and why others apply them. This works the notion of 'cultural scenario' too hard. It explains too little by trying to explain too much. A remedy to this dilemma is to recognize that culture is effect, not cause. It is Acholi experience of and response to a range of diseases that shapes their cultural scenarios, not the other way round. What the Acholi have learnt is that there are such things as epidemic diseases. Ebola and other epidemic diseases have caused the Acholi to elaborate segmented disease models, because Ebola and other epidemics do not fit the other models they have elaborated to explain other (non-epidemic) diseases.

We can apply the same thinking to the notion that funerals 'cause' Ebola in Upper West Africa. There is no doubt that processing the body of a dead person for burial is a major Ebola infection pathway. But to emphasize symbolic aspects at interment over techniques of body-handling results in flawed explanation. The cause of infection is washing the body – a technique of the body. Body-washing has ritualistic associations, but is primarily a practice associated with the work of the undertaker. It prepares the body for the funeral ceremony, much as one might prepare for a wedding by shaving or dressing nicely.

Nursing of the sick is an equally dangerous technique of the body, but would not so readily be described as a ritual. Insisting on rolling up body-handling processes under a single label – 'traditional ritual' – risks lopsided explanation, in which a continuous process – caring for the sick to the point of their final departure – is deemed purely practical in its first part but purely cultural in its second.

Insisting (as we ought) on a unified explanation for a continuous process reveals the problem. If it is stubborn to wash the dead then it is stubborn to nurse the sick. To insist otherwise blames the victim. Courageous refusal to abandon loved ones normally elicits admiration, not blame. So commentators on the Ebola epidemic, whether in Australia or elsewhere, ought to avoid stigmatizing West Africans for no other reason than that they care for their loved ones.

A better approach is to accept that rites are outcomes, not causes. Ebola prevention, whether involving the agency of local people or international responders, requires safer techniques of the body. But these techniques can be developed only by those who know what they are intended to achieve. 'Safe burial' as mandated by governments, and performed by trained and equipped teams from outside the community, splits apart technique and its social purpose. Better, therefore, to follow the approach suggested by local interlocutors – train us to do the safe burial, because then we can reintegrate burial within a wider social field.

If so, how could this be done? Techniques of the body serve an end. Neither a rite nor a technique stands on its own; both are embedded in a field of social relations and practices of social interaction. It is by addressing the dynamics of this social field that solutions to the dilemma of 'secret' and 'super-spreader' burials can be found. Better rites, and better technique, will result if the process of change is driven by societal considerations. But to get to a point where the practical implications of such an approach can be found, a journey is required, both through some aspects of social theory (in the remainder of this chapter) and through empirical evidence (the ethnographic details in Chapters 4 and 5).

Rites and techniques

Durkheim, Mauss and other members of the school of social science in France in the first half of the twentieth century, formed around the journal *Année sociologique*, saw clearly through some of the confusions and difficulties just outlined. To them, 'ritual' was group activity performed in a sacred register, not a cultural model, scenario or programme to be implemented. The rite was an expressive form of collective action serving to generate and recapitulate shared emotions. These feelings were then invested in sacred symbols.

Sacred symbols (totems) served as memory aids to rekindle group commitments, thus leading to the misapprehension that the symbols are causal. An observer of one of these ritual events might suppose that the flags, banners, pictures, masks and totems 'caused' the collective response. But this leaves out the fact that first the symbol had to be forged by investing it with group energy. Symbols are artefacts, and behind every artefact energizing techniques of the body can be discerned.

Durkheim's own work drew on early ethnographic accounts of Australian danced rites such as the corroboree.[6] From these accounts he came to understand that dance, as an expression of sacred ceremonial concerns, is not the implementation of a specific choreography; the choreography emerges from the dance. Where spontaneous dancing is based on schooled capacities for movement and gesture, patterned responses – specific styles – are likely to emerge. Durkheim's famous description of a corroboree perfectly captures the idea: 'passions so heated and so free from all control cannot but help spill over, from every side there is nothing but wild movements ... [but then] gestures and cries tend to fall into rhythm and regularity, and from there into songs and dances'.[7]

It would be truer in such cases to say that collective action assumes patterns, not that the pattern causes the action. The dance is entrainment, a capacity belonging to what has been termed 'the rhythmic brain'.[8]

Arguments imputing causal powers to cultural schemes have been extensively criticized by anthropologists of a Durkheimian persuasion.[9] In the Durkheimian account cultures, symbolic systems and institutions arise from collective action. Sometimes organization is an emergent property of spontaneous performance; in other cases it may be consciously planned. But in every case culture is the product of organization, not the other way round. The Durkheimians argued, with much evidence, that collective values and material transformation were 'co-produced'. As Durkheim and Mauss put it, the taxonomy of people is the taxonomy of things.[10]

The body was a unique reference point in the articulation of the world of people and things. At times, the body was marked or modified to convey this articulation. Group identity – conveying some messages about who could, or should, do what to whom – might literally be marked on the face in terms of scarification. Today we are more likely to do the same thing through clothes. But either way the body is an important medium for apprehending our organizational concerns.

And yet body science has been rather slow to develop, especially as an aspect of the social sciences. It was left to Marcel Mauss to explore the understanding that behind observably different techniques of the body are to be found different social contexts and modes of organization.

Understanding techniques of the body

Those who today read Mauss's seminal essay of 1935[11] might initially be a little disappointed. It seems little more than a list. But in seeking to be exhaustive it guides us to look at areas we might have missed. Fashion draws attention to itself, so we might have spotted the social significance of clothes without prompting. But would we so easily have paid attention to 'rubbing, washing, soaping', or cleaning of the teeth?

Mauss's paper was a manifesto. It itemized areas of attention. First in the list was sexual (gendered) division of techniques of the body (not only, he adds, division of labour by gender). Variation of techniques of the body with age, classification of techniques according to efficiency and transmission of techniques of the body by teaching and training round out his primary list.

He then gives a secondary list arranged according to the phases of life, and moments of the day. 'Techniques of adult life' start with 'techniques of sleep' which in typical Maussian manner he denies to be 'something natural'. He knew this was not the case because during the war he had learnt to trust his horse enough to risk the unnatural act of falling asleep in the saddle. A mountain climber, he had also taught himself to sleep when roped vertically.

Predictably there is a section on 'Techniques of care for the body: Rubbing, washing soaping'. The French (or rather the Gauls), he claims, perhaps rather dubiously, were the first to use soap. Doubtless, the British were rather late to get the habit. Mass-produced, affordable soap became common only after Lord Leverhulme devised a way to ship and process large amounts of palm oil from western Africa, and the bar of Sunlight soap was born. The date of the first emergence of 'native soap' made from the same ingredients (palm oil and ash) in the West African palm belt is unknown. It is not likely to be recent.

But Mauss is less interested in the origins of techniques of the body than in what we can learn from social variations in use. No technique of the body exists in a social vacuum. The point of his analysis is to establish that techniques of the body vary across social groups, countries and regions, and that these variations relate to differences in the way people are organized to perform mundane, universally necessary, activities in significantly different ways.

Everywhere people wash, but not everyone washes the same. Some go to the stream, others tip a bucket over their heads. In part, the variation is a matter of context (is there a stream?) and ancillary equipment (is there a bucket?).[12]

Ebola response offers an illustration. Safety protocols advise families waiting for an ambulance to set aside a drinking cup for the sole use of the patient, and to fill it by pouring, but not touching (see Chapter 6). But how many households have the necessary items to implement this advice?

An inventory of forest-edge villages close to where the first Ebola spillover occurred suggested that not every household owned a bucket.[13] Assigning to a single patient extended use of a cup might similarly tax some household equipment inventories. Shortage of containers is an aspect of extreme rural poverty making nonsense of 'safe nursing' protocols. So issues concerning *how* people wash their hands, handle soap, clean their teeth and drink are of great importance in addressing the infection threat from Ebola.

The mutuality of rites and techniques

There is more to Mauss's argument than simply to direct our attention to parts of social life we barely think about, such as who owns, or shares, a toothbrush.

The real point of his list of body technique is clear only when we return to the ways in which we classify people and things. I know one household (my own) where sharing a toothbrush and putting fresh paste on it are important signs that a marital quarrel reducing the parties to silence is about to be ended.

A funeral is an event rich in this kind of co-production; it addresses the technical problem of safely returning the body of the deceased to the ground, while at the same time resolving the social issues that the departure of the deceased has occasioned.

As will be shown in more detail later, an Ebola-mandated safe burial is problematic because in addressing a biosafety challenge it rides roughshod over the social issues. A funeral disposes of a corpse but it is also the occasion on which quarrels or debts are finally extinguished.

In rural Sierra Leone the partner will speak, in public, to the deceased wife or husband for one last time, with the onlookers, led by pastor or imam, urging that forgiveness be sought or offered. Perhaps more surprisingly, it is also a moment to settle outstanding debts: 'One person will enter the grave to receive the body sent down by two people. They will ask all present if the deceased has to pay anyone. If someone answers, the family will pay that person the amount owed. This debt must be settled before the person is buried.'[14]

To wash a corpse, to help dig a grave and to carry the corpse are important expressions of social obligations. To do one's duty brings about that indefinable quality of well-being known as 'blessing'. To try to evade such responsibilities risks social collapse, and being haunted by the spirit of the dead. For example, a youth leader angrily expressed concern that the spread of Ebola disease has introduced a very bad practice in their communities: 'We no longer do things in common. Even when your relative died, you do not see the body, neither the grave. We are not allowed to perform [a] ceremony, [and] we do not sympathize with others.'[15]

Banning funerals, we may infer, has destroyed social account-ability. Each pre-Ebola funeral proclaimed the importance of such accountability by setting up a bucket from which mourners could wash off the mud from the grave (unless they did so, further deaths would follow) and into which they threw a pebble to signify attendance.

Of course, there would be no way of knowing who had thrown which pebble, but the total number of pebbles would give the bereaved an ample token that they were not alone in their grief. The community had stood shoulder to shoulder, and the pebbles proclaimed it.

To disrupt this complex articulation of body technique and social life by abrupt and uncompensated material changes – to forbid washing, to impose cremation, to burn the grave cloth instead of giving it to the last child – throws the system of social dependencies out of balance at a moment of extreme vulnerability. Maussian theory indicates that ways need to be found to allow rites and techniques to co-evolve.

Washing the body

With the bucket safely arrived in the picture, we can now explore the scope of the technical field it heralds – namely, washing the body. This is one of Mauss's list of unexamined techniques of the body about which we might want to know more in comparative terms.

It will lead us towards the bugbear of Ebola response – washing of corpses.

Washing is a daily mundane activity. It helps us clean off the dirt and stress of work, and aids sleep. Small children, and very frail old people, are washed; others wash themselves, except if sick or injured, when (typically) marriage partners or very close companions will help.

The observer will quickly note quite a lot of variation in the modalities of washing, dependent on local resources and preferences. Variables include location and climate, whether the water comes to the house or a person washes at pump or stream, whether water is heated (something reflecting the availability of labour and fuel), and (in cases of ill health) on the type of sickness (the body may need to be steamed or cooled).

The field worker's notebooks are starting to fill.

Specific protocols and sub-routines for special body parts (for hair, eyes, teeth) will inevitably attract further attention, as will the vast array of ancillary technologies and specialist trades associated with washing. An army of craft producers prepares calabashes, buckets, 'sapo' (scrubbing materials) and soap, storage containers and drying materials, and builds shelter from the elements and screens for privacy, on and up to the plumbers and other specialists who sort out the en suite bathroom plumbing, piped water and blocked drains.

But little of this ancillary technology will make sense without first specifying the locally accepted or preferred body washing routines. I am of a generation in which British tourists had to have the concept and purpose of a bidet explained to them; even at that, usage outcomes might be quite variable.

Washing also attracts a vast array of secondary cultural attachments, none of which actually causes washing, unless your mother is exceptionally determined. This includes entire complex families of emotional and normative associations ('Johnny, you will wash your hands, or get no supper', 'you will sleep better if you wash first', 'cleanliness is next to godliness').

Furthermore, the student of technique, now thinking comparatively, will eventually conclude that the experience of washing is well nigh universal (except for maybe hermits and religious ascetics) and that it lasts a lifetime, and beyond.

Understandably, the desire to wash the body at death seems irresistible, to wipe away the signs of life's last struggles, and to prepare the corpse for its last journey. It is a natural reaction on the part of survivors, many of whom will have daily assisted the deceased to wash through the best part of a lifetime. It readily takes on symbolic or ritual associations. But the primary impulse is to wash the body for one last time. What could be more normal and practical?

This is borne out by the fact that we now know, from comparative anthropological work on Ebola, which highlights washing of corpses because it is a major infection pathway, that corpse-washing is found right across the African continent, and perhaps across the entire planet.

What the Hewletts write about body-washing among the Acholi would be very similar to what an ethnographer of the Mende in Upper West Africa might write. The Acholi are a Nilotic cattle-keeping people, the Mende of eastern Sierra Leone are forest rice planters, with hardly a cow to be seen, except on a butcher's hook. They are separated by a distance as great as the distance of London from Freetown. And yet accounts of Acholi and Mende washing of corpses are almost identical. This is not some kind of bizarre cultural ritual, as some Ebola responders seemed to imply, but a normal end to a human life.

Unsupervised learning

For Marcel Mauss techniques of the body were integral to the articulation of social and material life. The body was not just a tool of human performance, but also a tool for the generation, and regeneration, of social life. *How* the body articulates social and material dimensions of human existence bears further scrutiny. An example of this co-production of the social and material may help illuminate some of the specificities, as far as life in rural districts of Ebola-affected Upper West Africa is concerned.

Throughout the region the basic staple is rice. Households and communities are shaped around obtaining rice and eating it. In Mende thought, rice is synonymous with eating. I used to marvel at my research assistant, who ate every item of food on offer as we went on our daily survey rounds, and would then return home in the evening to say he had eaten nothing all day. He meant he had not yet eaten rice.

Closely observing how farmers select suitable rices enables us to trace out especially clearly the relation between techniques of the body and the cooperative social relations underpinning productive activity in a typical village community.

Some rices are deliberately introduced from elsewhere. They come with a recommendation, perhaps from a friend, community leader or merchant. In the language of neural network engineers, this is 'supervised learning'.[16] But West Africa also has its own rice – African rice. This is a distinct species (*Oryza glaberrima*), closely related, genetically, to a plant that grows wild in swamps and marshlands across the region. West Africans have gathered this wild rice for millennia.

Handling gathered grain led to spillage, and the rice planted itself around the homestead. Later, these handy patches of self-planted rice types were further selected for deliberate cultivation. The plant was changed by this selection into one better suited for farming. For example, selected types were less likely to shatter (lose seeds from the panicle) when handled for harvesting. A cultivar had been shaped by human practices. This was a product of unsupervised learning.

Later, the slave trade introduced rices from both East and South Asia. These were seed types which merchants, and even governments, had had a hand in promoting, thus products of supervised learning. But they grew alongside the local African rices, often in the same field, owing to mechanical mixing at harvest, and thus gene flow took place between products of both supervised and unsupervised learning. A number of distinctive farmer rice types began to emerge.

How were these farmer hybrids made? The available evidence suggests via crossing in farmers' fields.[17] For a spontaneous rice hybrid to arise there must be natural gene flow. Gene flow between rices is ten times higher in-field than between fields.[18] Thus for an inter-specific farmer hybrid African rice to emerge the African parent must be growing in the same field along with an Asian rice.

To understand these selection processes requires an account of the details of the techniques of the body deployed in rice seed harvesting and post-harvest processing, and how these activities are socially organized. Selection of seed for planting begins at harvest, and continues in storage (though rats may at times deselect what the farmer has reserved).

Who selects the seed to save? The rice harvest in a typical West African rice zone village is a distributed social event – it happens over a period, and the workforce varies. This is because the activity needs labour, but this is generally not paid, except in rice. The harvesting team will be mixed group of relatives, dependents and friends of the field owner (both men and women). The standard technique for harvesting deployed in many communities, even to this day, is to collect the panicles one by one, using a small knife, or sliver of sharpened bamboo. Reaping – bunch harvesting with a sickle – is found in some communities, but is a recent introduction.

Panicle harvesting allows off-types (rices that are morphologically different from the one planted) to be selected separately (and left in-field if not yet ripe). Off-types first survive selection at weeding, but only if the women of the farm (the experts in weeding) choose to leave them. I was once thrown out of a weeding party, because the women judged that as a man I was not percipient (or careful) enough to recognize immature rice among very similar grassy weeds.

Older food-insecure women, e.g. widows, often help with harvesting on the farm of a kinsman or in-law, and are rewarded by an allowance of what they harvest. Some might choose to involve themselves in sorting out the off-types that have been accidentally gathered into the bunches of rice waiting to be threshed. This is sometimes a necessary task since off-types may be harder to clean than the main variety. They might also choose to glean the freshly harvested field, and so keep any interesting off-types still ripening.

Thus the custodians of off-types are typically poorer, older, less strong women (and men) embedded within larger social units. Their existence becomes apparent from careful survey work on the composition of quarters, rather than through surveys of households, since many prefer to live independently, if they can. They comprise a class of farm helpers, rather than farmers, commanding less labour from others and with declining strength themselves.

If members of this group wish to plant rice for their own food security they have no capacity to fell the bush, or hire strong men as labourers. Thus they depend on 'borrowing' land that has already been cleared and cultivated, and is thus low in soil fertility. Such farmers are interested in any robust seed types that perform well on poor soil. In countries such as Sierra Leone and Guinea-Bissau, where farmer hybrids are particularly common, these rices have spread widely in areas of poor soils, or where other material constraints on farming have been experienced, such as isolation during times of war.[19]

What we get from this example is a sense of the manner in which techniques of the body, social organization and food security outcomes are co-produced. Particular configurations of body technique (e.g. panicle harvesting) and social values (e.g. opening up of spaces for widows to live independently, within the framework of the kin-group residential quarter rather than the household) go hand in hand. The specific forms of embodied technique, collective action and social organization have been co-produced, and largely through unsupervised learning. They are not consciously designed, but emerge through what people do.

Localizing burial

Understanding of the co-production of techniques of the body and forms of social life is essential for a grasp of the challenges posed by Ebola. These are both social and medical. Responders have not always fully appreciated this intimate connection. Preaching against funerals (arguing that the Ebola problem is driven by a stubborn adherence to cultural norms) is potentially counterproductive, since it fails to take account of the larger social field within which funeral techniques (or cultural practices more generally) are embedded. 'Safe burial' is the major case in point.

In Sierra Leone burial teams were (at first) recruited, trained and equipped in towns. Once problems with transport had been overcome, the teams often performed with skill, dedication and courage. But all burials had to be treated as Ebola burials, and the busy urban-based burial teams had no social connection with those they interred. By November 2014 Ebola responders had become aware that there was huge resentment of 'safe burial', and the WHO mandated a new approach, based on 'safe and respectful burial'. Religious leaders were attached to burial teams to lead prayers. But respect was an add-on, not integral to the co-production of techniques of the body and collective action.

A better approach would have been to embrace local participation, and to allow techniques and social meanings to co-evolve, as they did in the rice example discussed above. Collective action, social signification and safer techniques of the body would then march hand in hand. The argument is more fully elaborated in the following two chapers.

Conclusion

This chapter has outlined arguments for rejecting the idea that traditional culture caused Ebola Virus Disease to spread. Culture is epiphenomenal; it is a symptom, not a cause. Burials create pathways for virus spread, but so do several other, more mundane activities, not least practices of caring for the sick. So it is not helpful to distinguish ritual from practical aspects, and to invest the former with the sense of something exotic or bizarre. Both funerals and nursing are better viewed with a single explanatory lens – as techniques of the body. In turn, techniques of the body need to be understood as essential human resources in the co-production of material and social life. This provides us with a different analytical framework for assessing the problem of community Ebola response. In Chapters 4 and 5 it will be shown, by case study evidence from Sierra Leone, that where Ebola response initiatives – such as safe burial – were resisted or questioned this was not out of perverse adherence to tradition, but because imposed measures threatened the cooperative basis of social life. Communities argued strongly for training in safe burial, in order to adapt it to local social needs.[20] Understanding material and social co-production – it is suggested – is an important key to effective Ebola response.

Chapter 4

EBOLA IN RURAL SIERRA LEONE: A TECHNOGRAPHY

This chapter and the next offer an empirical analysis of the Ebola epidemic from the perspective of techniques of the body. They draw on a survey of twenty-six villages in central and eastern Sierra Leone undertaken in December 2014 at the peak of the epidemic. Topics discussed include local understanding of the causes of Ebola, access to treatment, local burial practices, and responses to quarantine and 'safe burial'. Findings show that villagers had formed their own evidence-based appraisals of links between techniques of the body and Ebola infection. It is also apparent that villagers had very negative views of the safe burial process. The need for this process was not denied, but community members demanded to be trained and equipped to carry it out themselves. Everywhere the call was the same: villagers needed to be able to invest the new techniques of the body to counter Ebola with appropriate social values. Following the argument developed in Chapter 3, a new co-production of body technique and local collective representations was required.

Exploring 'technique'

An initial requirement is to explain the use of the terms 'technique', 'technology', 'technography' and 'task group'. 'Technique' here refers to skill as an embodied set of social practices directed towards some kind of material or non-material end, with or without the use of tools and machines.

Marcel Mauss suggested regarding the body as our first tool. This may seem strange because technology studies often foreground instruments over the user of the instrument. Mauss's move is intended to provoke thought.

There is nothing contradictory about referring to the technique of a skilled singer. Human lungs and vocal cords are an embodied instrument. Nor, by referring to the body, or parts of the body, as an instrument, is Mauss retreating from the idea that technique always has a social context.

Social practice – the work of teachers, for example – is crucial in training the voice. To be self-taught is no exception, since the very idea of self-instruction implies pedagogy as a larger frame of reference. If we teach ourselves to sing we simply become teacher and pupil rolled into one.

'Technology' is used in the strict sense of 'knowledge of technique'. Properly, it should always be carefully qualified in terms of the domain of application.

Under the influence of commerce, advertising and journalism the word is often shorn of qualifiers, and used to imply something like 'our latest product'. When qualifiers are restored – 'new technology', 'advanced technology', 'smart technology' – hidden assumptions become apparent; the implication is that current knowledge of technique is inherently obsolescent, regressive or stupid. This is the language of advertising, and it is unfit for scientific purposes.

Technology is inadequately described unless contextual factors relating to usage are taken into account.[1] These contextual factors are inescapably social, and include all aspects of human cooperation, from familial intimacy to industrial division of labour. The centrality of the social in so-called 'new technology' is apparent in the now ubiquitous phrase 'social media'. The smartphone without contacts is not a phone.

'Technography' is a neologism, but useful nevertheless, because it immediately suggests a link with the more widely known word 'ethnography', used by anthropologists and others to index the detailed description of social processes, often based on directly observed qualitative data, including data derived from participation in, or being trained to perform, a task.

Technography focuses on the detailed description of technique, including descriptions based on the observer's acquisition of a specific technique, and is thus an important tool to acquire knowledge of technology. A title such as 'How I taught myself to sing: a technography' would make perfect sense.

Technography will also, often, provide information about the organization and performance of the 'task group'. Many techniques involve group effort, and group effort generally involves learning to work as a team. A full description of the task group, and how it is organized, trained and governed, is an essential aspect of technological knowledge. Research on task groups spreads over several fields, from anthropology to management studies. Two classic contributions might be mentioned – by Thomas McFeat and Frederick Brooks.[2]

Controlling Ebola requires new kinds of task groups to be organized and trained: barrier nursing specialists, safe refuse disposal groups, ambulance crews, safe burial teams. How these are formed and function, and relate to other relevant community groups, notably the family caring unit, should be a focus for reflection by anyone contemplating social mobilization for Ebola prevention.

Organizational style is also an important aspect of the study of task groups, and relates closely to the concerns of Mary Douglas and others with uncovering the 'elementary forms' that go towards making institutions work.[3]

McFeat opens his seminal book on the anthropology of task groups with an instructive story. As a young Canadian soldier, standing on the banks of the Ems river waiting to cross into Germany, in the last days of the Second World War, he saw a strange contraption on the river ahead of him. It was a segment of a Bailey bridge being floated across on pontoons, with four outboard engines strapped to the corners. A sergeant stood in the middle, trying to command the four motormen, in the teeth of a gale. Deafened by the wind, each motorman had his own ideas about when to apply power. The thing went round in circles.

Straight away McFeat realized that this was a boat designed by the army. It followed a parade-ground model of command. If the navy had been in charge, they would have built a lookout, blindfolded the four motormen, and connected them to the commander in the lookout by a system of pull-ropes and bells to issue unmistakable and unambiguous orders. The pontoon bridge section went round in circles because the wrong task group model had been applied.

The same question can be asked about Ebola control. Were new and often hastily improvised task groups for breaking chains of Ebola infection sound, both in regard to biosecurity objectives and also (crucially) in their fit with the local social context? Or did the response bring with it too many unquestioned assumptions on the part of responders about the way biosecure facilities and processes ought to be run in the social and medical conditions with which they were familiar?

The Hewletts report that local negative responses to patient isolation in previous Ebola outbreaks resulted from the use of tarpaulin walls in treatment units. This meant families could not see what was happening. Dark suspicions were formed. Sometimes, distrustful families reclaimed patients, and deadly consequences followed. This information was published in 2007, but still I saw several sites of (now disused) Ebola holding units and community care centres (CCCs) in Sierra Leone with opaque tarpaulin walls. Recurrently, informants complained that the inability to witness what was happening to their loved ones fed dark suspicions, and sometimes resulted in attempted rescues. Design of treatment facilities requires a social understanding of what needs to be witnessed, and why. A more thorough technography of care might support such better understanding.

Going home to be buried

Like McFeat, I begin with an observational vignette.

One day during a period of fieldwork in Mogbuama, a village in Kamajei chiefdom, a friend – an elderly hunter – arrived at my door. He had looked after me with great kindness for a number of years. A leading 'society' man, and headman of one of the village's five quarters, my friend's main complaint about me was the poor state of my Mende, since there were many things he would have liked to discuss with me more deeply.

He now struggled to explain that he had a daughter whom I had never met because she was married in a chiefdom some miles away, and that news had arrived to say she was sick, and close to death. She had TB. Would I help him by loaning my truck, then garaged at Njala, and drive to a village on the road to Moyamba, to collect the young woman, and bring her home?

Momentarily, I wondered about the advisability of transporting a very sick person on the back of an open truck, along a bone-shaking and dusty track. The last six miles would have to be by hammock, since my vehicle could not cross the two rivers that cut off Mogbuama, in those days, from the national road network. My friend assured me that 'yes, she must come', and 'yes, a hammock party would meet me' at the point where the footpath to Mogbuama joined the road.

When we arrived at the young woman's marital home it was already late in the evening. A party was waiting and silently arranged her, wrapped in what seemed to be several thick, locally woven country cloths, as comfortably as they could on the back of the truck, packing themselves and the items they needed around her, to provide shelter as far as possible from the night air. There were only whispered farewells, and few overt signs of the grief the husband's family must have felt at their loss. I was told to proceed.

We met the hammock team, silently waiting, as arranged. Relays of strong young men would take turns in managing the hammock along a rutted track, taking especial care over a long system of stick bridges carrying them over the braided and treacherous Tibai river, where it finally tumbled over the last step of the escarpment onto the coastal plain. Fortunately it was a moonlit night.

I waited a few moments while the hammock bearers and party of family and sympathizers moved off down the track, their way lit only by a couple of flickering storm lanterns. The procession reminded me of a poem by Robert Bridges, memorably set to music by Gustav Holst, about the funeral procession of a young woman, killed by grief, going to meet her dead lover.[4]

Hearing the music play in my head as I stood there in the moonlight blocked out for a time an obvious question. Why was this woman going away from her (living) husband to die and be buried at home?

Only much later did I begin to piece together the answer. It was complicated. Probably, there was going to be one last attempt to find a local cure, though, in fact, the young woman died the next day. As important was that she would now be laid to rest by members of her own family (*ndehun*, in Mende) in family ground. But I did not understand why the evidently distressed, not to say grief-stricken, husband did not play a greater part.

The explanation was that the marriage was one that in local social taxonomy is classed as 'incomplete'. This means that the promises of gifts and material help a husband and his family make to the family of the woman, before the union is agreed, had only been partly fulfilled. Until these obligations were fully met the man did not have the right to make arrangements to bury his wife. The body belonged to her *ndehun*. Only if he could afford, there and then, to discharge his obligations could he claim that right.

Behind this belongs a complex web of ideas about marriage, land and ancestral spirits. Landowning groups form alliances by marriage. Marriage, for Mende-speaking people, is a process, not a state. Only death determines whether, truly, you were married. A wife will sometimes answer the question 'are you married?' with the response 'time will tell'. The husband's obligations to the wife of his family are open ended. They have provided the greatest of all gifts – the means of life itself. This cannot be repaid, so the attempt is never ending.

But there is a ritual moment when enough has been provided, by way of loyalty to the woman's parents, for the parties to say this person is now truly our in-law; we are now sure he will never abandon our daughter, or us. This is when the marriage can be deemed socially to be complete. At death, the wife will then be buried where her husband chooses.

But going outside this contextual frame potentially stirs anger – the anger of a wife's family, of a soul not at peace, and of the ancestors. People fear a loss of blessing. The established order of social values has been affronted.

Of course, people also recognize that circumstances dictate that not everything can be done as required. A wife may die far from home and the burial has to be arranged *in situ*. But in such cases ritual transactions are needed to make reparation. A man can marry his wife after her decease, by offering what was not provided during her lifetime. This will regularize the situation, and thus calm the disturbed social (spiritual) forces. What is done is flexible. But something has to be done. Bodies cannot be dumped, but neither can they be buried where they are not supposed to be. Burial technique – and that includes Ebola 'safe burial' – cannot avoid adaptation to the social framework.

Care for the sick and dead

Chapter 5 describes in detail burial technique in rural Sierra Leone. First, some evidence on patterns of care for the sick and dead is presented and discussed.

Field study in Sierra Leone, carried out in December 2014, covered twenty-six villages (see Table 4.1). Selection was purposive. Twenty villages were chosen because they had been studied

Table 4.1 Whether or not to wait before seeking treatment for a sick villager (typical waiting times = 1–3 days)

Village	Ebola	Chiefdom	District	Road	Wait	Never	n =
1. Gbangba	Yes	Selenga	Bo	some	1	29	30
2. Gumahun-Faama	Yes	Badia	Bo	some	0	25	25
3. Bawuya	Yes	Kori	Moyamba	none	18	7	25
4. Fogbo	Yes	Kori	Moyamba	none	19	8	27*
5. Moyamba Junction	Yes	Fakuniya	Moyamba	good	16	14	30
6. Peri Fefewabu	Yes	Gaura	Kenema	some	8	22	30
7. Komende-Luyama	Yes	Lower Bambara	Kenema	good	3	22	25
8. Baima	No	Gbo	Bo	good	3	27	30
9. Mogibisi	No	Gbo	Bo	some	4	21	25
10. Mokebie	No	Gbo	Bo	some	0	22	22
11. Fengehun	No	Kakua	Bo	some	1	28	29
12. Gbumbeh	No	Kakua	Bo	some	2	28	30
13. Sarguehun	No	Kakua	Bo	some	4	24	28
14. Njagbema	No	Kamajei	Moyamba	none	17	13	30
15. Mobaiwa	No	Kamajei	Moyamba	none	15	15	30
16. Mogbuama	No	Kamajei	Moyamba	some	17	13	30
17. Foindu	No	Yoni	Tonkolili	some	9	21	30
18. Masengbeh	No	Yoni	Tonkolili	none	22	8	30
19. Maraka	No	Yoni	Tonkolili	none	22	6	28
20. Bo	No	Gaura	Kenema	none	1	17	18
21. Jagbema	No	Gaura	Kenema	some	5	25	30
22. Njala	No	Gaura	Kenema	none	1	25	26
23. Sanola	No	Gaura	Kenema	some	4	18	22
24. Senehun Buima	No	Gaura	Kenema	some	7	22	29
25. Mapuma	No	Koya	Kenema	some	13	17	30
26. Belebu	No	Tunkia	Kenema	some	11	19	30
TOTAL					223	496	719
Per cent					31%	69%	100%

* 3 missing values, names in bold = Ebola cases

previously, and baseline data existed. Only one of these villages had experienced an Ebola outbreak, so six more villages with Ebola cases were added to the sample.

Seven villages with Ebola cases out of a sample of twenty-six over-represents the true community-level incidence of the disease, which is about one in forty villages, given a rough total of 16,000 village communities in Sierra Leone.[5]

The research design selected a range of rural communities along a transect stretching from the Gola forest on the Liberian border, through Kenema District (Eastern Province), and Bo and Moyamba districts (Southern Province), to Tonkolili District in central-northern Sierra Leone. Most villages were Mende-speaking, but villages in Tonkolili District spoke Temne. Mende and Temne are the two main languages in rural Sierra Leone, in addition to Krio, widely spoken as a national lingua franca. There are some significant cultural differences between Mende and Temne communities, especially in regard to burial practices.

The material discussed below relates to three groups of villages. The first group comprised villages adjacent to the boundary between the northern and southern provinces, where there was an outbreak of Ebola in July/August centred on the village of Fogbo (Kori chiefdom), as briefly discussed in Chapter 2. This outbreak preceded the international response surge in the last three months of 2014. The second group comprises villages without Ebola cases in the general vicinity of the Fogbo outbreak, and served as a control. For one of these villages (Mogbuama) baseline data exist from 1983.[6] The third group comprises villages in Kenema District in the east, adjacent to the Gola Rain Forest National Park, Sierra Leone's last area of undisturbed tropical rainforest. Two of these villages experienced Ebola outbreaks in October/November 2014, and showed some evidence of the impact of the international response. Other (non-Ebola) villages were examined because of their closeness to the forest edge, thus illuminating potential problems of inaccessibility.

Figure 4.1 Villages in Tonkolili, Moyamba, Bo and Kenema districts surveyed as part of an Ebola impact study

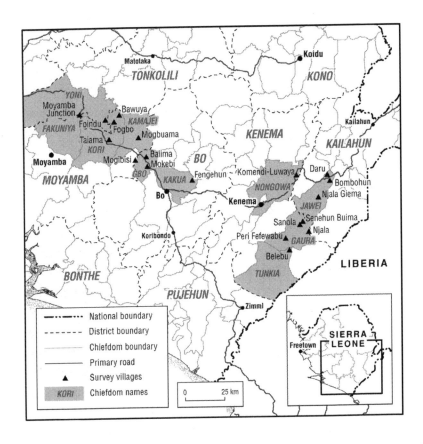

Methods included a mix of quantitative and qualitative data-gathering techniques. A questionnaire was designed to elicit information from a random sample of around thirty adults per village (half of whom were female) on responses to sickness, including presumed causes of Ebola. Focus groups were organized to allow different groups of villagers (male elders, female elders, and youth – both male and female) to discuss a range of open-ended topics including causes of sickness and death, quarantine, normal ways of preparing corpses for burial, reactions to 'safe burial', ways of funding visits to health centres and other forms of medical care, and access to Ebola ambulances.[7]

When possible, the different focus groups were run simultaneously, to guarantee independence of viewpoint. Facilitators were trained to motivate discussions by moving from general to particular prompts. For instance, groups were asked to discuss common recent instances of sickness before any discussion of Ebola took place. Groups were encouraged to establish their own agenda of topics for discussion. Each group had a second facilitator to monitor side comments and body language.

Interventions were managed through a numbered card system. Each speaker traded in a card before making her or his point. This allowed coders to enter information on the types of person speaking, and the number of times they spoke, without compromising the anonymity of the speaker. All those answering questionnaires and participating in focus groups provided informed consent, and all personal names relating to victims, survivors and so forth were reduced to initials to preserve the anonymity of human subjects.

Descriptive analysis was undertaken based on tabulation of questionnaire responses, transcription and coding of focus group responses, comparison of responses for villages with and without Ebola, and assessment of intra-village variation, by gender and social seniority.

Village perspectives

What people thought caused Ebola

In the questionnaire survey two related questions were posed at different points in the interview:

Q. 1 What do you understand to be the causes of this sickness?

Q. 2 What is your own idea about how this disease spreads?

The first question was framed in general terms to avoid any imputation that the survey was checking up on the reception of Ebola messages. Nevertheless, respondents appear to have played safe, and said what they thought they were expected to say. But the second question differs, in that there is now a specific prompt. The interviewee is explicitly asked to say what he or she thinks.

This results in a clear shift in the balance of responses, and is here understood as evidence that people formed their own conclusions about causes, independent of messages received. Answers couched in terms of bushmeat significantly decline. Prominence is given to a new answer – that body contact is a key factor in spread of infection.[8]

Data relating to answers to the two questions were then examined for three Ebola village samples and four matched controls (see Table 4.2). Of the control villages, two were accessible by vehicle along farm access roads (Foindu and Mogbuama) and two (Mobai and Njagbema) were accessible only by footpath. About

Table 4.2 What people thought caused Ebola

Causes of Ebola as understood in general (Q. 1)

	Males	Females
Bush meat a cause	51	39
Bush meat not a cause	52	63

Causes of Ebola as understood by respondent (Q. 2)

	Males	Females
Bush meat a cause	12	10
Bush meat not a cause	91	92

Cross tabulation of answers to Q. 1 and 2

	Q. 1	Q. 2
Bush meat a cause	90	22
Bush meat not a cause	115	183

half of all males and 40 per cent of all females gave the answer that bushmeat was a major cause of Ebola infection in answer to Q. 1. This reduced to about 10 per cent when people were asked for their own understandings.[9]

There are no clear differences between communities with direct and indirect experience of Ebola. In both cases around 90 per cent of all villagers discounted bushmeat as a significant transmission pathway when describing their own beliefs about Ebola, and instead emphasize risk factors such as touching infected bodies. In other words, where public messaging concerning Ebola risks was wrong, as in the case of bushmeat, it was rejected in favour of risk factors with better empirical grounding in local experience.

The questionnaire also invited respondents to pose questions to the research team. These questions frequently implied scepticism about bushmeat as an infection pathway; for instance: 'we have been eating bush meat for a very long time and have not experienced this disease, why only now?'.[10] But despite this widespread scepticism many people, in fact, refrained from eating bushmeat, and saw this as something for which they should be compensated by the Ebola response; '[since] we have been asked not to eat bushmeat, then provide for us' was one such blunt response.

It is also worth paying some attention to the 'don't know' or 'no answer' responses (see Table 4.3). Fifteen women and twenty-one men provided answers of this sort, comprising 17.6 per cent of all answers, but 25.9 per cent of answers in communities with Ebola cases.[11] It seems strange that lack of awareness of the causes of

Table 4.3 Negative ('don't know' and 'no answer') and positive responses for villages with and without Ebola cases

	Ebola village	Non-Ebola village
Negative answers	22	14
Positive answers	63	106

Ebola would be higher in villages with direct experience of the disease. These data may signal heightened distrust and a purposeful refusal to express a view.

It is relevant to note that twelve negative ('don't know' and 'no answer') answers came from people aged over sixty (one third of the total). Older people are more likely to be elders of the powerful sodalities, Poro and Sande. Sodality funeral practices have been implicated in Ebola transmission. The Fogbo outbreak was one such instance. Negative answers may suggest, therefore, the workings of sodality disciplines of secrecy rather than reflecting a poor state of factual knowledge concerning Ebola transmission pathways. This flags an issue, further addressed in Chapter 6, about the role of the sodalities in social mobilization against Ebola.

Access to treatment

The first requirement in an Ebola outbreak is to isolate confirmed Ebola cases in a special facility where palliative care can be safely administered. Hospitals unfamiliar with the necessary biosafety requirements spread the disease in the early stages of the epidemic, resulting in many deaths among medical staff, and dedicated Ebola Treatment Centres (ETCs) were established by agencies such as Médecins sans frontières to reduce nosocomial infection risks.

The disease moved across Sierra Leone from east to west, and then to the north-west. For a time, before the surge of international assistance in late 2014, ETCs were overwhelmed with demand, and sometimes turned patients away. Some patients were bussed long distance from newer infection areas in the west to longer-established facilities in the east, where case numbers were beginning to decline.

As a result of these long-distance movements of Ebola victims, families and patients became separated, and reporting of patient progress and outcomes to families was imperfect. Rumours spread about the alleged purpose of ETCs – to harvest body parts – and Ebola victims tried to avoid being taken to treatment centres. Some sought help from traditional healers (herbalists). The flight of these patients into the countryside reduced chances of survival, but increased the chances of new clusters of infection emerging.[12]

With the surge in international response, provision of beds began to catch up with need. New local holding and treatment centres (community care centres [CCCs]) were established at chiefdom and district level, and proved to be effective and acceptable.[13] Communities were often positive about CCCs (despite the reservations of many responders) because they offered palliative care, free feeding (taken as evidence of goodwill) and after-care reintegration packages for survivors.

Even though staffed by volunteers with limited medical expertise, or even none at all, these centres did not become, as some had predicted, motors for the spread of the disease. There were few reports of staff infections, for example. The free care and feeding marked out the centres from previous healthcare provision. And because centres were local, families could keep an eye on loved ones, and follow outcomes. Most communities said they wanted such facilities repurposed rather than removed, once Ebola had gone. Clearly, they helped reduce fear, and increased local knowledge of the true nature of the disease.

The field study reported here was undertaken in December when many community care centres were still being built, especially in the north, where the epidemic was most actively spreading (see Figure 2.5 in Chapter 2). This was too early to assess their impact, but even so a key question could still be posed. Spread of Ebola would be reduced, and patient survival chances increased, if patients reported early (within the dry phase, generally lasting three days). So what, in general, influenced the speed with which villagers reported diseases to the health authorities?

In the questionnaire survey a random sample of fifteen male and fifteen female adults in twenty-six villages (see Table 4.1)[14] was asked whether they ever hesitated to send a sick person to a health centre, and if so, by how many days they would delay for different classes of patient (children, adults and older people), and why. The three parallel focus groups in each of the villages were also asked to discuss access, finance and other obstacles to early reporting.

Of 719 persons interviewed 223 (just under a third) reported that they would wait for between one to three days to find out how the sickness progressed. In effect, they would sit out part or most of the dry phase of Ebola. With the onset of the wet phase it is too late to move a patient safely, except in a specialist ambulance, manned by a crew with protective clothing. Not all villages, of course, had roads, and hammocks would be the only alternative, at least as far as the roadhead. Hammock carriers have no protective clothing.

Data on waiting times were examined against a ranking of local road conditions. The aim was to ascertain whether prior experience of Ebola and poor road conditions influenced reporting times (see Table 4.4). No evidence was found that prior experience of Ebola reduced the chances of sending sick persons promptly for treatment, but poor road conditions did have a significant effect.

Did prior experience of Ebola make a difference in moving the sick? In villages without Ebola cases 33 per cent of persons said they would delay seeking help by one to three days or more. In villages with Ebola cases 37 per cent of persons said they would delay seeking help by three days or more (Table 4.4).

Table 4.4 Whether experience of Ebola cases and lack of road access reduce chances of patients moving to medical care

	Move	No move
Ebola	105 (110.27) [0.25]	62 (56.73) [0.49]
No Ebola	276 (270.73) [0.1]	134 (139.27) [0.2]

	Move	No move
No road access	99 (134.99) [9.6]	115 (79.01) [16.39]
Some road access	282 (246.01) [5.27]	108 (143.99) [9]

Did road access make a difference to delay in moving the sick? In eight villages with no road access 52 per cent of persons interviewed would wait up to three days or more before seeking medical help. In eighteen villages with (some) road access only 22 per cent of persons would delay seeking help by three days or more (Table 4.4).

Note that the three Ebola-affected villages in the Fogbo outbreak (Fogbo, Bawuya and Moyamba Junction) all had a high likelihood of persons not moving immediately for medical assistance. However, the same was also true of three control villages without Ebola in neighbouring Kamajei chiefdom (see Table 4.1). Note also that Moyamba Junction has very good road communications; high waiting times cannot be a reflection of poor road conditions in this specific case.

How were delays explained?

When asked directly about their personal experience ('had they ever been too sick to seek help outside the village?') nine people in Bawuya, a small off-road village infected with Ebola from the Fogbo outbreak, answered 'yes'. Lack of money and quarantine restrictions were the major reasons given.

This set of answers included all three Ebola survivors in Bawuya. In earlier answers, two of these survivors described being treated in an Ebola Treatment Centre (ETC). The final stage of both these journeys was in an Ebola ambulance. Thus these answers might be taken to imply that reaching an ETC might not have been the original intention, but a decision taken for them by the authorities.

Interviewees were then asked, in the case that a member of their household had a fever, which of three statements was more likely to be true: take them to a hospital immediately, wait for some time to see whether they get better, or never take them to a hospital. As noted above, early reporting of Ebola cases is crucial to improved chances of survival. Only seven respondents said they would act immediately. Seventeen would wait.[15]

People were also asked how long they would wait if the case involved a child, an adult or an old person. Respondents provided estimates in terms of days or fractions of days they would spend waiting. For a child the waiting time ranged from one hour to seven days (average = 1.2 days). For an adult the time was longer, ranging from one to eight days (average for adults = 2.1, average for older people = 2.0).

Reasons were given to explain these differences. Children, it was frequently suggested, were weaker than adults, and could die more quickly. Views on older people were split. Some thought that they should be taken for treatment as soon as possible, but one respondent reckoned on a delay by a day for a child, three days for an adult, and a week for an older person, bluntly commenting that 'old people are always sick'. Another person thought there should be no difference between children, adults and the elderly ('all are humans'). Even so, this respondent would wait a full day before seeking help.

In Fogbo, the decision to wait before seeking medical help was reported by seventeen interviewees. Average waiting times before seeking medical help were similar for both children and adults (children 1.1 and adults 1.0 days), but somewhat longer for older people (2.1 days).

Lack of money was offered as a reason to delay in two cases. Once again one person openly voiced the idea that older people are 'always sick', and that it was impossible to respond to every case. The somewhat longer waiting times in Bawuya, compared to Fogbo, probably reflect the fact that Bawuya is three hours' walking distance from medical treatment in Taiama, whereas Fogbo has its own medical post.

For comparison, it is interesting to look at focus group results for Bo-Gaura, an off-road forest-edge village on the margins of the Gola forest in the east of country. The account was pieced together from comments made by members of all three focus groups, and provides a graphic picture of what medical evacuation, for Ebola, or any other disease, would entail in these remote and isolated conditions:

> [The] road is not motorable and people use hammocks to carry people to health facilities at a distance. Travelling is mostly at night, [and there are] lots of hills in this community.
>
> Most of the bridges are made of wood, [are] not strong, and you get hungry when trying [hard] with the hammock.
>
> Money is needed, for support to young men, [this includes] provision of torchlight for night travel, and rain gear for travelling during the raining season.
>
> [If such movement is needed] a family meeting will be summoned and every one [is] asked to contribute money to pay for transportation and treatment fee, and to 'beg' [i.e. motivate the] youths to transport [a] sick person in [the] hammock to the nearest health centre.
>
> Family members are taxed, married children are asked to pay some amount, and youths are begged to carry the sick if the road is not accessible by vehicle or bike.[16]

Off-road villages maintain hammocks for emergencies of necessity, and young men are skilled in transporting sick people in them. Hammock travel is a specific technique of the body with its own hazards.

> [The] hammock swings, [so there is risk that the] carrier will contract sickness from [an Ebola] patient.

Bo-Gaura had had no Ebola cases, so this remark is evidence that villagers were able 'to think like epidemiologists', in inferring potential infection risks for a disease not yet experienced directly.

If treatment is needed in a health centre outside the village cost issues become major constraints. Money is needed both for the hammock ride, or to charter a motorbike taxi, and then to pay for medication, treatment and feeding. A night-time or rainy-season ride is an especially expensive proposition, since the evacuation team will also need torches and/or rain gear. It is not hard to understand why villagers with few or no savings hesitate to rush for medical treatment.

> [My] son was treated at home not in hospital because money was not available. He was given local herbs to drink.[17]

> [To move a sick person] we will use motorbikes and it will cost Le 15,000 [about $3.00, or about a day's wages for a farm labourer] from Peri to Joru health centre [a distance of about five kilometres]. [The decision to move a person will be taken by] the chief and family members. For a stranger, the *hotakei* [lit. stranger father, landlord] will decide on carrying the sick person. [If there is no money] the family member, town's people and the person accommodating the stranger will contribute to pay the money. If the money contributed is not enough, we will pledge the person's plantation or property to pay the money.[18]

> Sick people are taken to Fogbo or Taiama by hammock or okada [motorcycle taxi], where hospitals are available.[19]

> Family members will inform the chief, who in turn will inform the youth leader [*Ndakpo mahei*, literally 'chief of the age mates']. The hammock will be used and youths given a small token as motivation.

In Mogbisi, Gbo chiefdom, Bo District, female elders offered the following description of how care for the sick is organized (see tabulated responses in Table 4.5). A husband, wife or older child will take charge of the nursing. For a woman the carers will be members of her own lineage (*ndehun*). For wives born outside the village (see below) this implies either moving the patient back home, or that a person from the home village will move to the sick woman's marital

Table 4.5 Comments on care, by female elders of Mogbisi, Gbo chiefdom

Who cares for seriously sick persons?	*'If a man, he will be cared for by his wife and eldest son, if a woman by the daughter.'*
Who cares for an adult woman when sick?	*'The relatives from the family of the sick person. Sometimes her peer group.'*
If a man or woman has no husband or wife who cares for him or her?	*'The relatives of either side, or [if a] stranger, the host.'*
If the sickness cannot be cared for in the village, what arrangement will send the sick person to a hospital or health centre in [an] other location?	*'The chief and the family will gather the community to loan money from within the community or club (osusu) for medication.'*
If there is no money to carry the sick [person] what will happen?	*'The family will loan or sell their land and plantation.'*

location to offer care. In cases of Ebola such mobility could be a factor in inter-village spread of the disease.

Serious sickness generally involves arranging a loan, pledging of tree crops or selling of land (see comments of the youth focus group in Peri Fefewabu above). The link between recurrent sickness and endemic impoverishment is a long-term feature of agrarian poverty in rural Sierra Leone.[20]

Calling for help

The National Ebola Response Commission established a telephone 'hotline' ('117') to process requests for burial and evacuation of sick persons by ambulance. After initial problems the helpline scaled up, and appears to have worked quite well in urban and peri-urban areas of Freetown and the main provincial towns, from which (in the end) a large proportion of Ebola cases came.

Western Area – greater Freetown – alone accounted for about 40 per cent of all confirmed Ebola cases. However, the helpline suffered from the incomplete national cell phone coverage (only about 70 per cent of the country) and the difficulties routinely experienced in rural areas of keeping mobile phones charged. Charging phones is a thriving cottage industry for owners of small generators in many larger villages, but is not easily afforded by all. Many phones need to be charged once an emergency arises, adding to response times.

Figure 4.2 shows these blank spots. Coverage gaps are especially significant in Koinadugu District. Owing to its isolation this district had few Ebola cases overall, but there was an important outbreak in Neini chiefdom, an alluvial gold mining area at the centre of the district, with no cell phone coverage.

Figure 4.2 National cell phone coverage at October 2014

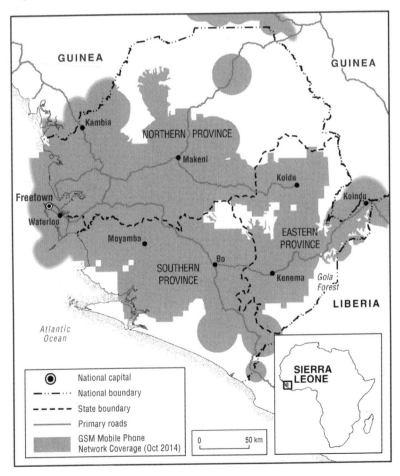

A communications gap around the margins of the Gola forest should also be noted. This is hilly terrain, and even when coverage is indicated, villagers often need to seek higher ground to get a signal. Peri Fefewabu – an outbreak village – is one such place. Lack of phone coverage in an area at risk of zoonotic spillover might be a serious issue if outbreaks were to recur.

Movement of the body at death

The likelihood of bodies travelling home in pre-Ebola times has been indicated in the fieldwork vignette above. Such movements were especially likely for women, for reasons already indicated, or for the bodies of urban residents who had maintained a strong identity with their rural home (typically, first-generation migrants).

Many males wanted their bodies to be repatriated to be close to the focus of family life. A publicly known place of burial is especially important where the family has rights to land or chieftaincy. In recent times, grave sites have taken on an increased importance with the rising value of rural land for agricultural investment. In a patrilineal community, repatriated male bodies help guard the land rights of descendants of deceased persons.

In the case of a wife, the husband has to give an account to the family of the cause and circumstances of death. He will fight hard to get the body of his wife home, not least to dispel any suspicion among her family that the woman died of mistreatment or neglect.

A need to move the body is not only confined to urban migrants. Rural–rural movement is also likely at death, especially where the deceased person had the socio-legal status of a stranger (*hota*, in Mende).

Strangers are recognized in customary law as persons living outside their chiefdom (or sometimes village) of birth. A survey of three villages in Kamajei chiefdom in early 2014 offers evidence of the typical proportions of village populations classed as strangers (from 25 to 40 per cent).

About one third of all residents of the three villages recorded in Table 4.6 were classed as strangers. One quarter to one third of this stranger group was male. Thus the bodies of about 8–10 per cent (0.33 x 0.25, or x 0.33) of male village residents are liable to be taken home after death. But it will also be noted from Table 4.6 that about two-thirds to three-quarters of all strangers are women. This is because many rural women (typically 40–50 per cent) marry outside their home villages. Rural marriage in Sierra Leone is predominantly virilocal (i.e. the woman moves to her husband's home village). Whether the body of the wife is then buried in the husband's village or the woman's home depends (as noted) on the status of the marriage payment.

Many village marriage payments remain incomplete for years. Farming life is hazardous, and farmers are in the grip of poverty.

Table 4.6

a) Stranger origins in 3 villages in Kamajei chiefdom, 2014

	Households	Total population (2014)	Hota (born outside village)	% of all adults	Female hota	% of all adult hota
Mobai	53	348	60	25.2	46	76.7
Mogbuama	99	590	179	40.4	110	61.5
Njagbahun	60	446	101	31.2	71	70.3

b) Rates of marriage completion, 3 villages in Kamajei, 2014

	Married females as % of all females in sample	A. Stranger females, complete marriages	B. Stranger females, incomplete marriages	C. Citizen females, complete marriages	D. Citizen females, incomplete marriages
Mobai	51.1	1	12	0	11
Mogbuama	86.8	6	14	3	10
Njagbahun	52.4	0	11	0	10
	62.2	15.9% (A/A+B)	84.1% (B/A+B)	8.8% (C/C+D)	91.2% (D/C+D)

Promises to the family of a farmer's wife may have to be deferred owing to misfortune and lack of resources. The wife's body will be reclaimed by her family unless debts are quickly settled post-mortem.

Any such post-mortem movement was forbidden by emergency regulations covering the Ebola epidemic in Sierra Leone, and all burials, irrespective of cause, were (supposedly) carried out as rapidly as possible by 'safe burial' teams. But this represented a large legacy of 'incorrect' burials. How this legacy will be dealt with in the post-Ebola era remains to be seen. There might be some pressure for reburial. A basic requirement under Ebola regulations for 'safe burials' is for these to be properly documented. Failure to address the reasons for 'home' burial might have lasting adverse consequences for rural land tenure arrangements and social cohesion.

BURIAL TECHNIQUE

International responders at times talked about infection chains sustained by 'stubborn' villagers persisting in 'hiding' corpses and engaging in 'secret' burials. Thus it was important to find out more about normal burial practices, and why people felt aggrieved at not being able to follow their expected procedures. Fieldwork was carried out in December 2014 involving parallel focus groups for male and female elders and young men and women, in the hope of encouraging all age groups to talk as freely as possible about Ebola, and especially issues relating to burial technique, since this was an important point of friction and misunderstanding between Ebola responders and affected communities.

The ethnographic detail on burial technique is extensive. It is perhaps sufficient here to consider just two villages, Fogbo and Foindu. These are chosen because they are located on the main ethno-linguistic divide in the country, and had some direct experience of the disease. The Temne- and Mende-speaking communities in Sierra Leone are each estimated, in total, to comprise about 40 per cent of the national population, and by repute have different burial customs.

Care needs to be taken to avoid ethnic essentialization. The idea that fixed ethnic or linguistic affiliation drives burial practices is a further example of the doubtful notion that culture is causal. To draw on an example given by Mauss, the French and English troops in the Great War of 1914–18 used different shovels, and dug differently, because they had developed different practices on different kinds of land, not because they belonged to different nationalities.

The Yoni Temne of Foindu and the Kpa Mende of Fogbo share a common environment of grassland interspersed with patches of bush and riverine forest. There is considerable intermarriage across the border separating them, though more often Temne men marry Mende women, giving them access to more abundant land on the Mende side of the provincial divide. Many people along the border speak both languages fluently. Thus we perhaps ought to expect a continuum of beliefs and practices, not a sharp break.

In fact, the continuum is not entirely smooth. In former times, the boundary was militarily contested between the Temne polity of Yoni and the Kpa Mende state, with a major military concentration at Teyama (Taiama). A large river (the Teye) separates, rather than joins, the two groups. Although Foindu and Fogbo are only a few kilometres apart on the right and left banks of the Teye there is no significant river traffic between the two places.

Transportation and administration take the people of the two villages in different directions. Fogbo people take their major medical cases to Moyamba or Bo (Southern Province), while Foindu people seek medical assistance in Magburaka or Makeni (Northern Province).

Fogbo: a Kpa Mende village

Appendix 1 (see page 153) shows transcripts of segments of parallel focus group sessions held for male and female elders, and a mixed gender group of young people in Fogbo, a village in Kori chiefdom hit by an Ebola outbreak in July/August 2014. These were the first cases in Moyamba District.

In all three groups informants were prompted to talk about the process of handling the body from death to interment. These responses refer to 'normal' burial processes (i.e. what would have obtained prior to the requirement for compulsory 'safe burial').

The youth group provided a short, generic account, but covering the activities in which they would be involved, namely transfer of the corpse to the grave, and some details of the layout of the grave itself, which they would have helped to prepare.

The women elders spoke more times, but concretely, apparently about the burial of a specific person, without elaborating much on their largely factual answers.

The male elders group, by contrast, not only described specific techniques of body management in some detail, but also provided important interpretive insights on symbolic aspects, such as the fact that when the corpse is being washed in the backyard of the dead person's house the head needs to be positioned towards the sun (the presumed direction of travel of the soul) or the soul will be disoriented, and remain on earth, tormenting family members.

The details about the inverted bucket placed where the feet rested when the body was washed are also informative, since it is stated that the soil under the bucket will be used to rub on the body of the wife or husband, to *separate the living from the dead, so that the dead will have no power to inflict pain or bad luck on remaining family members.* This seems a potential infection pathway for Ebola. In some cases a trench is dug under the washing platform to drain away the water, since this is thought to carry risk of infection.

In Bawuya, a small settlement close to Fogbo, the focus group for young people added that *if it is the first time the wife/husband lost a partner, the remaining [partner] is washed ceremonially with part of the grave soil [and] water to avert bad luck/misfortune from the remaining partner.*[1]

Both male and female elders in Fogbo describe the grave cloth given to the last child to wash in the stream and then keep. The men add moving detail about the river washing out and carrying away the soil from the grave, indicating the end of life, as the soil is carried away by the river. Presumably this cloth is a potential Ebola infection hazard, and should, under current rules, be burnt. WHO protocols for safe and dignified burial[2] recognize that families will want to offer prayers at the grave, from a distance. But this is a static provision. There is no scope for an excursion to the river, and its poignant associations are lost as a result of Ebola restrictions.

Foindu: a Temne village

As a Temne-speaking farming village of about the same-size (population c. 500) a few kilometres upstream on the Teye river on the opposite (right) bank, and administratively located in Yoni chiefdom, Tonkolili District, Northern Province, Foindu is a good comparative foil for Fogbo. Foindu did not experience Ebola directly, whereas Fogbo did.

Male elders described what they knew of the Ebola 'safe burial' process: *According to information, it involves placing the corpse in a plastic bag, spraying of the house, putting the corpse in the ambulance and taking it to the burial site – one pit for several bodies (ten and over)*. Another informant said there was no other option: *washing the body and dressing for burial is preferred, but we have no choice, so [we] accept government's recommendation*. However, the group also requested to be trained for the work: *Let the community be given the protective gear and advice so we can undertake the burial.*

The normal burial process was then described, but rather briefly, with a stress on religious aspects: *Previously [we] send a message to all families, then [a] meeting [is called] where the following is decided: [how to] provide food at home, [and] wash the body. Men wash men, women wash women.* Moving the body around, for washing and for burying, is important information, because body-handling is bound to be a risky process in cases of Ebola death: *bulky women are carried by men, [but] small[er] women can be carried by their women folk and back to the house (by hand).* Then *youths go and dig [the] grave,* prayers are said over the dead, and the corpse is transported to the grave, which has been fitted in advance with an internal structure of board and sticks. The soil is then placed on the body after further prayers have been said.

When a wife dies, first it is required to *report [the death] to [her] family and ask what should be done. The family grants permission to do the burial according to [her] religion.* The husband is *asked to bless, [and] forgive,* and the imam offers general *duwao [Arabic] asking for mercy.* If the death was caused by sickness then *sorcery [divination?] is done to find out the cause of the illness.*

Female elders in Foindu provided specific information on procedures applied at the moment of death. *First close the eyes of the dead person, [done] by the one who had being helping or taking care while she was sick. Also the mouth is closed.* Both actions would pose an infection hazard in an Ebola case.

Then the body is moved from the bed, to prepare for washing, *by two women, excluding those who have been helping,* thus adding to the number of women at risk of cross-infection.

As many as six people take the dead for washing. Three wash her with white cloth, [satin] gloves, [and] hot water; if [she is] a Muslim zakat is given out from the cups of water, out of every ten cups of water one is left as zakat.

The corpse is then placed *on a board and undressed by three women, who wash the corpse in a Muslim way by means of janaba. The washing of the corpse starts from the right hand from the head to the feet, then [turns to] the left side. Those washing the corpse first under-take the alwala.*

The grave-digging is always done by men. They volunteer for the work to secure blessing. The workmen share tools: *The same pickaxe and shovel are used by all.* Further light is shed on the grave itself: *Some graves have rooms where the corpse is placed and some do not.*

In agreement with other groups, young people in Foindu objected to the way 'safe burial' was carried out. *No, we don't like it. [The] dead should be buried with honor and respect. Empower [the] community to bury our dead with full traditional rights; train us to perform the burial process.*

Foindu youth offered much detail when it came to the burial process, as it used to be, before introduction of Ebola restrictions.

When one is dead, female or male, family members will cry on the body, hold or touching the dead. After which the oldest of the family will inform the chief of the death. Chief then gives permission for the body to be prepared for burial.[3]

The potentially hazardous task of closing eyes and mouth is presented in a new light. People speak about severe sickness as being a time for the disclosure of hidden matters. Confession in such circumstances is thought to be advisable, even healthy. A woman with a difficult pregnancy may be told to confess the names of clandestine lovers. But the secrets of those close to death are handled with greater discretion. *The eyes and mouth are closed by the wife or husband, or by the eldest child, because the person should be mature enough to keep the secrets of the dead.*[4]

A summary of the burial process in Foindu compiled from comments by the three groups is set out in Appendix 2 (see page 155).

For a wider regional perspective on burial technique it is useful to compare information on Fogbo and Foindu with findings from a small village close to the Liberian border. Bo-Gaura is on the edge of the Gola forest reserve in Sembehun Section, Gaura chiefdom. It has no road, but is reached along a rutted, rock-strewn footpath. Techniques of the body deployed in undertaking in Bo-Gaura are essentially the same as those described for both Foindu and Fogbo, in the centre of the country.

The following account is compiled from remarks supplied by male elders:

The body is laid straight, eyes and mouth are closed and cloth spread over the body. The body is moved from the bed to the mat by four people. The place for washing the body is prepared at the back of the house. [This] is fenced with tarpaulin or mat and a hole dug where water will drain. Two pairs of gloves are given to the washing people. One scrubs the skin with soap and sapo [scrubbing material] and the other pours water. After washing the body, it is moved from the wet mat to a dry mat. The people who washed the body are responsible for dressing it. The person's fine[est] dress is put on [the body] which is later wrapped in white satin and sprayed with perfume. Four young men are charged with the responsibility to take the corpse back home. The body is laid on a wooden coffin and taken to the house where it is officially handed over to the religious leader. Six youths take the body to the mosque and place it outside the mosque. Prayer is offered on the corpse and [it is] later taken to the grave.[5]

Sodality burial

Elders from Gbo chiefdom, in Bo District, offered some comments on sodality burial (see Appendix 3, page 156). The details are confidential and were not disclosed in the focus groups meetings. Sodality funerals are secret events – not 'secret burials' in the sense implied by Ebola responders, but closed events restricted only to members of the sodality.

Village-level concerns with 'safe burial'

Teams of mainly younger people from urban areas were trained to carry out 'safe burial', equipped with transport, personal protective equipment (PPE) and chlorine sprays. With town-based vehicles in short supply, teams were at first slow to respond to calls for safe burial in more distant, inaccessible settlements such as Fogbo. It took burial teams four to five days to reach Bawuya to deal with the dead bodies of people infected by the Fogbo outbreak. In October 2014 Kenema District had only one burial team for the entire district, and it was heavily overstretched. Failure to reach suspected Ebola deaths after several days generally resulted in villagers burying the corpse as they saw fit.

Whether out of fear or pressure of work, burial teams appear, sometimes, to have used inappropriate methods:

The way they throw the corpses into the grave is the thing that I hate about the burial. These people cannot lay the corpse gently, but throw it. They don't even wash the corpse, nor dress it respectfully.[6]

[The] dead are not handled with care and respect; male and female are [both] buried by male burial team; it is wrong: instead of holding the body, sticks are used to push dead bodies on to the stretcher.[7]

At times, rather than negotiate with uncooperative villagers, hard-pressed burial teams resorted to threats. In Peri Fefewabu (Gaura chiefdom) a rumour that chlorine spray was deadly appears to owe its origins to threats of this sort. *They put fear into us and ... were making threatening remarks. They said 'we are spraying chlorine so that people will die'; The husband of the lady who first died of the disease [after attending a funeral in Liberia] survived and is still alive, but when they sprayed the chlorine, more people died.*[8]

In other cases, burial teams carried out a dangerous job in difficult circumstances, and several villagers acknowledged it was a necessary task, and that team members were placing themselves at risk. The teams appear to have taken good care of their own safety. According to interviews in Bo with burial team personnel and management in December 2014 no cases of infection among the teams had been reported up to that time. Team members were, however, shunned by neighbours, and some were asked to leave their accommodation.

Villagers also took note that burial teams did not become infected, but this served to reinforce their conviction that they, too, could be trained to do the work.

We have seen [that] since the burial team [members] have been in this process none of them has been infected. We want the government to provide the protective gear used by the burial team so that we can bury the corpse without being infected.[9]

Disquiet at the work of burial teams was widely expressed across the sample. Since 'safe burial' applies to all deaths, whether of Ebola or not, then most if not all villages in Sierra Leone have by now experienced the work of the burial teams. The idea of villagers being trained and equipped to take over the work was raised without prompting in nearly a quarter of all focus group sessions. In settlements with Ebola cases this proportion rose to half.

The opinions expressed by focus groups in Baiima, Gbo chiefdom, and Foindu, summarized in Appendix 4 (see page 156), are typical of the larger data set.

A burial team perspective

Local responders – burial teams and contact tracers – came in for a lot of criticism from community members, but did a difficult and dangerous job with considerable commitment. Their viewpoint should also be represented.

A burial team manager[10] reported that:

It is true there are areas we cannot get to easily because of bad terrain and no coverage for mobile phones. We were over-stretched with few personnel in the burial teams, and very bad vehicles/burial vans. Command was scattered and [it was] difficult to locate who [needed us] and when. However [improvements are coming] with a command centre and coordinator. More vans have been provided. The workload has been divided. Now we have [agency name deleted] doing some burial, and areas of operation have been allotted, with more burial teams [deployed?] [Thus] the response is better these days compared to before. [But we need to] restrict movement to ease Ebola. With regards to cooperation and collaboration much improvement is [needed] ahead. On stigmatization: all I know [is that] my boys are stigmatized. Some say they are doing better this time. I also recommend that people change their perceptions of the burial teams, as [team members] are at risk. But none of them has [yet] been affected with Ebola. I recommend in the future to build [special] quarters to accommodate them.

A contact tracing officer[11] commented on the muddle of mixed messaging that had derailed some of the response effort, and on evident problems with quarantine. He also connected the hazard posed by corpse-washing with the far from dignified nature of safe burial:

> They said [Ebola] has no cure. This is why people [were] not going to the clinics/hospitals in the country. But now people are saying there is a cure. [This has] made the people to completely doubt the medical team [owing to mixed messages]. Let them use the [surviving] victims [to] talk to people; many are afraid. What is going wrong in the quarantined home is that food is not sufficient and some go around in the bush to seek for wood [firewood] and condiments. People can accept survivors if they possess discharge certificates and can be observed for another twenty-one days. The reason Ebola is still in the country is that people wash dead bodies before the arrival of the burial teams, and they [the teams] do not give dignified handling of the corpse as well as burial. It is true that members of the burial team are stigmatized as well as doctors and nurses. People are washing dead bodies, and [there is still] mass movement in and out of the villages and cities.

Undertaking

Calls to train community-based burial teams were loud and insistent. So why did this call fail to elicit a prompt response? Part of the problem was logistics. It was easier and quicker to mobilize and train teams at central locations, rather than in a distributed manner in communities. But part of the problem seems also to have been the way modern life 'invents' areas of ignorance concerning practical and necessary activities that have become thoroughly professionalized.[12]

WHO[13] counselled empathy in regard to Ebola burial, but on what practical experience of burial was that empathy to be based?

As a child, on the backstreets of a Lancashire mill town, I lived opposite an undertaker's premises, and thus had some familiarity with its daily routines – the power saw whining as boards for another coffin were cut to size, the comings and goings of the large black hearse, my grandfather standing to attention and taking off his hat when a newly filled coffin left the chapel of rest. I had no fear of (or ghoulish interest in) the corpses resting on the premises overnight; it was a family business, these were our neighbours, and to my five-year-old mind everything seemed perfectly normal.

But any such awareness of the daily routines of death has rapidly declined in developed countries. I would be hard pushed to know where I could now relive my childhood experiences. Since the nineteenth century body-handling at death has been professionalized, and then rationalized. In Britain, according to a fascinating study of the sociology of undertaking by Brian Parsons[14] – the author himself by background an undertaker – the family undertaker largely disappeared at the end of the twentieth century owing to corporate rationalization.

Funeral directors' premises may retain the external trappings of a family business offering a personalized service, but many are now part of large chains. The body may be taken to a local chapel of rest in the first instance, but is likely soon to be on its way in an unmarked refrigerated van around the urban ringway to a centralized cold store. Only once arrangements are in place for the funeral service, days or perhaps weeks later, will the body, now doubtless barcoded for track-and-trace monitoring, make its last and perhaps rather lengthy journey to a local place of cremation.

Parsons summarizes the story as follows:

A shift in ownership of funeral firms has occurred especially during the last three decades as independent organizations have been acquired by large organizations. This latter type of firm ... exploited occupational control attributable to the rationalization of the death and disposal environment by managing their funeral operations on a centralized basis, thus achieving cost savings ... a number of negative consequences are apparent ... there is no evidence that [operational economies] are passed on to the consumer ... retention of the original trading name deceives the public ... [and] a degree of depersonalization exists.[15]

In short, undertaking has been industrialized, and escapes the everyday notice of the layperson in modern settings. Only the ritual of a funeral remains visible. It is perhaps not surprising that Ebola responders – many from backgrounds of the sort just described – tended to see funerals in Sierra Leone in terms only of 'traditional ritual', and missed the importance of training communities to transform body-handling technique, since this was part of the funeral process with which they had little or no direct experience.

As a result, procedures of body processing were misread as if they were rites, and judged strange, as if a proverbial visitor from Mars had stumbled across a broken-down white van full of frozen corpses in transit along a London ring road and had concluded the locals had a passion for necromantic joyriding.

Because local family-based body-processing techniques were also dangerous, by reason of Ebola risk, some responders concluded rather too quickly that West Africans were deliberately putting themselves, and the world, in danger through their stubborn persistence in performing traditional cultural rites.[16]

The problem was compounded by the seamless way in which local people, carrying out their own deeply felt responsibilities to the dead, wove together actions and meanings in their burial processes. The meanings arise from the actions, and are for this reason not easily separable. The grave cloth is muddied by the soil from the grave, and given as a keepsake to a child, who rushes in tears to the river to wash it, and the soil disappears down the stream as surely as the stream of the deceased person's consciousness had ebbed away. The cloth, cleaned and dried, lives on as bedding for the child, and a tangible last link with a departed loved one. Action, materiality and signification are one.

Quarantine as technique

When an Ebola case is confirmed the patient is isolated, and high-risk contacts – basically people in the same household unit as the person with Ebola – are quarantined for twenty-one days. If there are subsequent cases, households are further quarantined, until the infection chain ends. The issue of how quarantine was applied, and by whom, and how it varied in urban and rural areas, is complex, and a fuller account requires further investigation. These comments, then, are provisional.

In Sierra Leone, quarantine was at times enforced by the security services (the army and police). Incidents of violence, of the kind experienced at West Point in Monrovia, seem to have been rather rare.[17] In some cases, security personnel may have preferred not to grapple at close quarters with infected persons.

In a follow-up study undertaken in August 2015, in Peri Fefewabu, a village adjacent to the Gola forest, south of Kenema, where there were fourteen cases of Ebola in October 2104, we were told that close contacts of Ebola victims were quarantined in classrooms of the local primary school. Like many such premises, the primary school is on the outskirts of the settlement, separated from the dwelling area. The police and army maintained a cordon around the school, but sanctions on those attempting to break quarantine were imposed by local chiefs in the form of fines, and not by physical force.

In fact, the people of Peri praised the security services, since they had helped in bringing food, water and firewood to quarantined persons. The chiefs, we were told, used discretion in sanctioning quarantine breaches. Wanton breaches were fined, but not where delivery of emergency rations by Ebola responders was late or unforthcoming.

Some might say that this less draconian approach risked further spread of Ebola. Others might argue, however, that it helped establish that quarantine was a 'commonsense' measure. In effect, chiefly understanding of a basic human need for food might have facilitated a more general local acceptance of quarantine, honoured (in this case) in the breach. It is also worth adding that the Peri outbreak, like all other village outbreaks in the region, quickly came to an end. As will be shown in Chapter 6, local efforts in imposing quarantine and preventing unnecessary inter-village mobility had a significant impact on epidemic outcomes.

In part, these local efforts were successful because quarantine was not an alien idea to villagers. Enquiries uncovered numerous cases of public-spirited self-quarantine, undertaken to protect family, friends and neighbours. Focus group discussants pointed out that quarantine had been widely adopted by villagers to deal with disease threats such as smallpox in the past, and that the practice was still maintained to address 'goat plague' (PPR, *peste des petits ruminants*), a viral disease of sheep and goats in which infection occurs through contact with body fluids of infected animals, and which presents a useful model for thinking about Ebola.

Villagers are often aware (see focus group evidence collated in Appendix 5, page 157–8) that unless measures are undertaken to quarantine sick goats – sometimes by adopting strict community bye-laws – a village might easily lose all its goats. Furthermore, PPR, like Ebola, is an emergent disease in Sierra Leone, since it was introduced from other parts of Africa in the post-civil-war period, as a result of poorly managed animal restocking programmes.

Although by and large quarantine was rather readily accepted, this does not mean that villagers were satisfied with the way quarantine was managed. Some sensed, in particular, that responders made up the rules as they went along, and that they had not always thought through their protocols very thoroughly.

In Peri Fefewabu villagers were quick to comment on an inconsistency. Responders said there should be no home care, and that close family contacts should thus be isolated in the school, with each contact family group occupying one classroom. But nothing had been said about what should happen if one of the close contacts fell sick, other than to ring '117' (in an area of little or no cell phone coverage!). Slow, or no, response by '117' would in effect mean the household group was administering home care to an Ebola patient unaided, but now in a school classroom, without even the limited affordances that the home could provide. How was this reducing the infection risk, they wanted to know.

Villagers were also aware of, and confused by, some apparent bickering between different response agencies about the quarantine rules to be followed. There seemed to have been no agreed, general quarantine protocol among responders as late as October/November 2014.

There were also concerns about how close contacts, and indeed households, were defined. The frequently adopted 'cooking pot' definition of a household was probably the most relevant, in that the family feeding together probably organizes a lot of basic care of sick members together. Thereafter difficulty sets in, since 'households' (defined in this sense) do not map readily on to houses. Many buildings have two or more households within them. Some members of the same household may live apart, in separate buildings.

The international responders were directed in identifying people to be quarantined by their contact tracers, some of whom were perhaps too young and inexperienced for this kind of work. These contact tracers might be born in the village in question, and were available for work because schools had been closed. Typically they were at secondary school, perhaps in a nearby town. Their knowledge of precise, up-to-date sleeping arrangements might have been far from perfect. In some cases, finger-pointing may have owed more to local disputes than to Ebola exposure. Villagers in Peri Fefewabu implied that not all those exposed were quarantined, and not all those quarantined had been exposed.[18]

Again, the conclusion the villagers drew from this was that they should have been given the responsibility to design and implement their own quarantine rules, perhaps based on a revival of the old separation arrangements for smallpox victims. Every family has a farmhouse in the annual rice farm, and it is often an alternative place of residence for the nuclear family during the busy part of the farming season. It might have been better to organize isolation of Ebola patients in temporary shelters built near to farmhouses, as was the case with smallpox and other infectious diseases, than to use the local school. It would have been better to be quarantined close to a good source of food, water and fuel, to reduce the motive to break quarantine. The school was a choice reflecting the convenience, or lack of local knowledge, of external responders.

Actual quarantine breaches deserve closer study. They tend to be seen by responders as antisocial acts born of selfishness or ignorance. An Ebola infection chain in Sierra Leone in July/August 2015 stemmed from a quarantine breach by a man in his mid-twenties, living in Freetown. He 'absconded' at the end of Ramadan to be with his family in a village in Kholifah Rowalla chiefdom, Tonkolili District. In the daily bulletins of the National Ebola Response Commission, however, it is reported that he had a job in the city and was in the habit of returning to his village each month to bring his family food and money. He infected his uncle, who had taken charge of caring for the young man when he became sick. The mother's brother is in effect a second father in the social conditions of rural Sierra Leone. An alleged moral 'breach', therefore, becomes on closer examination a picture of social responsibility and moral rectitude. The gap between social and medical norms is abundantly apparent.

Survivors

As of 23 August 2015, 28,041 people in Guinea, Liberia and Sierra Leone had been infected with Ebola, but 16,739 persons (59.7 per cent) had survived. Survival rates improved as rates of detection and availability of early palliative care improved. Survivors themselves contributed to this positive effect.

Survivors have two important embodied skills. They cannot be reinfected, so can safely touch and care for Ebola victims, and can be trained to do much of the work needed in Ebola care centres. Secondly, they provide tangible, living proof that the disease can be overcome. Ebola is not a death sentence. Accordingly, survivors have been used to spread positive messages about Ebola treatment, especially the message that early detection and admission greatly improve survival chances, as well as reducing risks to others.

However, survivors have suffered a degree of stigma, and some have been shunned by their communities. A particular problem is that the virus survives in semen, breast milk and the eyes for much longer than in blood or other body fluids. Survivors can convey the infection through sex or breastfeeding for many months after they have recovered from the disease. It is still not fully known how long this period lasts, or what risk of infection it poses. In particular, mixed messages about the period of sexual abstinence have proved confusing. Reintegration of survivors thus presents a range of unresolved challenges.

The following accounts provide a sense of what the disease does to its victims, and the problems they face. But these accounts also emphasize how survival is an opportunity to help others confront the disease.

I know Ebola is a dreadful disease because it has claimed the lives of my mother and [my] son (aged seven years). Ebola is caused by *tombu* [an entity which burrows inside the body] which cannot be seen with the eyes. We can contract [it] by contact with dead bodies, urine, faeces, sweat, blood, and through the eyes, cuts, and sperm from sexual intercourse. [In] my own case, [my sister and I] contracted it from my late mother who became ill a few days from return[ing] from a burial of one of our family members. She did not disclose how she contracted it until her death [probably this was revealed on the mother's deathbed]. We were isolated when her result came in later, of Ebola. We were confused, stressed and isolated from the rest of our neighbours with whom we stay. We were quarantined with minimal food, [and with] police officers around with guns, which made us more depressed. Later, samples of blood [were taken], and the result was positive. I refused eating as the three of us were taken to the treatment centre at Bandajuma [MSF] camp. It was a miracle we were discharged and we are at home and feeling better, only that people in the neighbourhood do not visit us, even though we are all declared Ebola free ... The food is not sufficient, and we have lost all our properties [clothes, bedding, furniture] because of Ebola – they were burnt. The good part is that we are free from any further outbreak for now, but the bad part is how can we recover our lost glory. I recommend that the government use all the victims on social interaction and health talk, to people who are in doubt [about] Ebola.[19]

I developed fever, with loss of appetite, vomiting and frequent stool. I thought of Ebola, because our mother died of it. At the treatment centre I summoned up courage and accepted conservative treatment. The good thing about the centre was that any food requested was provided. [After] a few days our brother died, which made us discouraged. I had sleepless nights, although I continued with the fluids, drinks, drugs taken, until miraculously I recovered. One day we were told Ebola has been conquered in our bodies, and we are to be discharged ... The good thing of the treatment centre is that they encourage us – that is, the health personnel, and drugs and food were provided. [There were] counsellors around. Bad things [are that] we should have been provided with music and spiritual support. After discharge they should encourage the community we are living in for acceptance; [and] continue to educate the communities of affected victims to pay visits to them and not to isolate them. They should use us on social counselling of affected victims.[20]

Querying Ebola from the forest edge

The questionnaire interviews ended, according to our field team's standard practice, by asking persons interviewed if they had questions of their own they would want the interviewer to write down and report. Many people availed themselves of the opportunity, and the questions they posed offer a fascinating insight into debates typical of what might be termed a village university of 'people's science'. Some of the confusions and contradictions of Ebola response are firmly nailed, with, at times, a quite delightful sense of irony and rhetoric.

The questions set out in Appendix 6 (see page 159) are especially worth pondering, since they reveal, for a set of communities with few if any roads and surrounded by the bats and monkeys presumed to be vectors of Ebola, some of the basic contradictions associated with the Upper West African epidemic.

Moreover, focus groups did not just discuss Ebola. They were also encouraged to talk about a range of other medical problems, to develop a sense of where Ebola sits in the larger picture of health concerns. Many groups commented on the neglect of other major diseases, notably malaria, owing to the national preoccupation with Ebola.

Men also often chose to talk about hernia. This is a major problem in farming communities heavily dependent on hand labour. A health system more oriented towards thinking in terms of techniques of the body, as Ebola now demands, might pay closer attention to hernia. The view of the male elders in Foindu was particularly explicit. It was, they said, a disease of 'hard work' and 'poverty'. Treatment, ruinously expensive by village standards, was 'by surgery, costing Le 1,500,000 at Makeni, plus vehicle charter – Le 200,000, or travel by transport vehicle – Le 50,000'. Deaths were reported. One man, without money for treatment, had suffered stomach pain for ten years, and was unable to walk. Deaths eventuated.

Convergence: thinking like an epidemiologist, and like a villager

Infection numbers began to level off, and then to fall, in the first affected districts of eastern Sierra Leone, from October 2014. A key factor was better survival rates. This depended on an important shift in medical perception – that the disease was more like cholera. Implementing best practice palliative care, to the highest standard, with a strong focus on rehydration, was said to be the key.[21]

It was at this point that some convergence became apparent between the thinking of international responders and affected communities. Simple messages configured around body technique underpinned home-care protocols – drink oral rehydration solution, or coconut water, nurse at a distance, only the patient handles the cup, one person only to be nominated as the caregiver, visitors and sympathizers to keep their distance.

Local skill and determination doubtless played a part in bringing about this shift. In evidence to be discussed in Chapter 6 one paramount chief trained and equipped his own locally based burial teams, and there was a rapid and significant reduction in further local spread of the disease.

Stories also began to emerge concerning attempts to improvise protective items from locally available materials such as plastic bags. One such improviser was a colleague, Roland Suluku, who made an Ebola 'suit' from cheap plastic sheeting. Commonsense application of basic knowledge concerning infection risks and rehydration requirements, plus determination, allowed some family members to pull through, where emergency calls for help went unanswered.

Such achievements, it transpired, were not unprecedented occurrences. Hewlett and Hewlett[22] document how one woman in

Gulu, northern Uganda, force-fed several members of her family on liquids and brought them through the 2000 epidemic. A young Liberian nursing student took a similar approach with three members of her own family, in this case attaching drips, and saving three of them. She protected herself through improvising protection with bin liners.[23]

Perhaps the most compelling evidence that villagers had begun to think like epidemiologists is to be found in the large appetite, evidenced above, for community-level training in safe burial. The message conveyed by these insistent demands is that the infection risks posed by burial had been accepted and understood. Help us now to beat the disease, was the gist of this local cry.

Bearing the risks of Ebola and the isolation of some forest-edge villages in mind, one female elder in Senehun Buima posed an exceptionally provocative question:

> I'm a traditional birth attendant, we have pregnant women in our village. If it happens someone wants to put to bed [give birth] and we do not have medical equipment but local materials, how can we manage, because government says we should protect ourselves?

Clearly, the questioner implies, the authorities can stop burial, but they cannot stop birth. So the question conveys its own answer – more needs to be done to provide better *in situ* capacity to protect against Ebola infection. As will be shown in Chapter 6 this was not an impractical demand, even if more could and should have been done to support it.

But to travel down this path, even if only part of the way, implies international responders also made progress towards understanding the integration of village practices and social realities.

There is some evidence that a shift in this regard occurred as the epidemic in Sierra Leone approached its peak. By September 2014 WHO had included some home-care advice in its social

Figure 5.1 'Taking care of someone with suspected Ebola: be safe while you wait'

Taking Care of Someone with Suspected

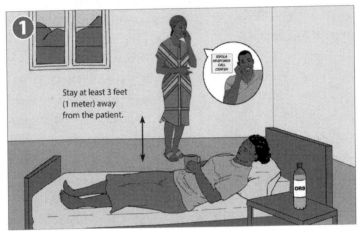

Stay at least 3 feet (1 meter) away from the patient.

If a loved one is sick with suspected Ebola, call 117 for help. Do not touch them, their blood, or their body fluids (vomit, feces, urine, sweat). Tell them to drink plenty of Oral Rehydration Solution (ORS) or water. Patients who drink lots of ORS early have a much better chance of surviving.

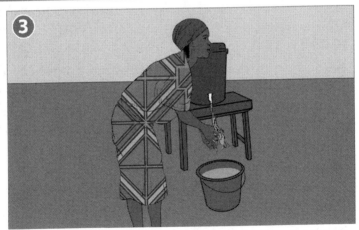

When caring for a sick loved one, do not touch them, and wash your hands often with soap and water or chlorine solution, even if you haven't touched them. Wear a protective barrier such as gloves and cover all uncovered skin. Wash your hands every time you provide care.

U.S. Centers for Disease Control and Prevention

Ebola: Be Safe While You Wait

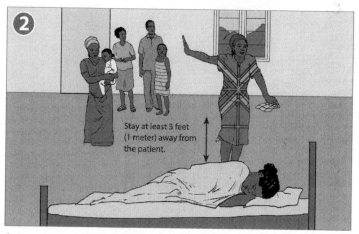

Stay at least 3 feet
(1 meter) away from
the patient.

Only one person should care for the patient while you wait for help to arrive. Do not let other family members come close or provide care. Stay at least 3 feet (1 meter) away from the patient. Do not touch the cup the patient drinks from. Refill the bottle without touching it. Do not touch the bedclothes, sheets, or other items the patient has touched while sick.

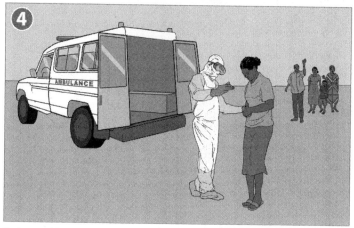

Patients with suspected Ebola should be cared for in a treatment facility. If you have a sick loved one, they have the best chance of surviving with medical care at a treatment facility. This helps to protect your family too.

mobilization prospectus, even while also stating plainly (and contradictorily) that such care was to be avoided. In November, six months into the epidemic in Sierra Leone, the Centers for Disease Control and Prevention (CDC) produced a poster entitled 'Taking care of someone with suspected Ebola: be safe while you wait'.

By entitling the poster 'Be safe while you wait' its designers cleverly avoided any clash between the medical mantra that there must be no home care and acceptance that some cases would receive help only after a long wait, or perhaps never. This, surely, is evidence that some epidemiologists were beginning to think like villagers, even if medical orthodoxy instructed them otherwise.

Equally, there is clear evidence of convergence from below. Foindu youths were either very attentive to the latest messages, or good at working things out for themselves, for they were aware of recommendations concerning one-on-one nursing and the use of bin liners even as that advice first began to circulate.

In mid-December 2014, only a matter of weeks after the CDC poster was issued, these young people summed up the process for the benefit of the Njala team:

> The infected person is placed in a house by him/herself while other members are moved away. An elder of the family is appointed to provide care for this individual, through the use of black plastic bags to protect face, hands and feet from coming into contact with individual. This individual provides encouragement, support for the infected [person] until taken to the hospital. This elder may be very close family member (father, mother, child, sister or brother).[24]

Conclusion

Experience sooner or later persuaded local opinion that Ebola was a disease of body contact, and populations at risk began serious re-evaluation of techniques of the body associated with nursing the sick and burying the dead. Although passing on instructions was extensively adopted as a means of aligning local opinion with epidemiological viewpoints, in the expectation that information would drive behaviour, this chapter has presented some evidence that local ideas changed independently of the loudhailers. So much was happening at once, as the epidemic peaked, and the international surge kicked in, that it is hard to be certain about cause and effect. But there are several pieces of evidence to suggest some significant changes were driven from within. Perhaps one of the most secure facts, in this regard, is that provided by the young woman in Bo-Gaura, who remarked that a lurching hammock and a vomiting patient might be an infection risk for hammock carriers. I know of no messaging that mentioned hammocks as an infection risk, or that even acknowledged the existence of this most necessary item of village emergency medical kit, so this remark, surely, is an example of a villager understanding the implications of the disease within a context of local practices and social arrangements. There is evidence, also, that local people were proactive in reinforcing quarantine, in imposing movement restrictions, and in improvising protection to reduce risk of infection when handling Ebola cases. But above all there was a widely shared grassroots view that safe burial was something that communities could and should have been trained and equipped to undertake for themselves. This conviction ran quite against the grain of epidemic management thinking by external responders, in which the two words – 'home care' – were difficult to utter. So an issue arises, to be addressed in Chapter 6, about whether there was more scope for local agency than was at first assumed, and if so, how this aspect of Ebola response might have been better supported. In short, this final chapter will assess the hypothesis that local common sense helped end the epidemic.

COMMUNITY RESPONSES TO EBOLA

Ebola control is predicated upon six key factors: identification of the virus, extraction of the patient, application of safe nursing techniques, tracing and quarantining of close contacts, and safe burial. A major issue for epidemic control was whether or not communities could change their approach to care of the sick and burial of the dead. This meant the population had to rethink familiar and established techniques of the body – in both nursing and in handling the dead – to prevent transmission of the virus.

Addressing the first three factors depended in large part on resources brought by the international Ebola response. These included mobile laboratories, testing procedures, telephonic and transport equipment to report cases and safely transport patients, and purpose-built Ebola treatment units, and medical and logistical personnel to deploy these items. The tracing and quarantining of contacts and safe burial, however, raise a large number of social issues. The international response did not bring, by and large, personnel or resources to deal with social issues, since these are often highly contextual.

For Sierra Leone, UK Aid recruited British National Health Service volunteers, and units from the British army. The Americans and French governments did likewise in Liberia and Guinea. Such people had transferable skills, and could learn quickly and train others in how to address the biosafety, logistical and human security aspects of the epidemic. It would not, however, have made much sense to bring volunteers from the UK Department of Social Security (for example), because expertise in the management of social issues depends on local knowledge. So a question was how was this local knowledge to be mobilized.

Social mobilization was needed to create an environment in which biosafety control measure would be accepted and enhanced. Was there expertise to address these kinds of social challenges? The social sciences are less strongly supported relative to other areas of scientific knowledge formation globally, but especially in Africa, where sometimes politicians equate social investigation with political opposition. Much necessary social knowledge is locked up in the heads and practices of people in communities, and remains largely undocumented. Perhaps nowhere was this more true (as pointed out above) than in the case of burial. How, then, given a dearth of documented, evidence-based information, was a social response to Ebola to be organized?

Given that Ebola was a new disease in the region it was assumed by those coordinating the response that a priority would be to supply information. International responders displayed little confidence in the capacity of local populations to learn quickly about biosafety risks for themselves. This chapter will argue that too much emphasis at the outset of epidemic response was placed on messaging. However, the international responders were ignorant of how an epidemic of Ebola would play out, since this was the first time such an event had occurred. Some of the messaging was wrong, and undermined the confidence of communities in what they were being told. More attention, it will be argued, might usefully have been paid to the concept of local knowledge, and specifically the question of how experience is formed in the face of unprecedented circumstances. In this regard, the scholarly community, where a large part of writing on the region has been dominated by anthropologists, historians and others trained in the tradition of the humanities, was not well set up to support the Ebola response, having for the most part operated on the basis that local knowledge was cultural knowledge, in the sense defined by Geertz.[1] People's science was not its strongest suit.

The present chapter will suggest that in the event there was an effective community push-back against Ebola, based not on culture but on a capacity for rapid evidence-based local learning. This was in effect a people's science of Ebola control, and depended on assessing biosafety risks freed from prior cultural assumptions. The purpose of the chapter is to suggest that this local empiricism was a significant factor in ending the epidemic, to explore how it worked, and to propose that agencies charged with coordinating Ebola response should in future more fully embrace the possibility of rapid local evidence-based learning, and figure it into their thinking about epidemic control.

Messaging: a false start?

In September 2014, as the big international push against Ebola got under way, WHO produced a document entitled 'Key messages for social mobilization and community engagement in intense transmission areas'. This set the agenda for Ebola control based on what the document calls 'the messaging approach'.

This approach, the document explained, is 'driven by the need to be empathetic, action oriented (promoting specific preventive behaviors) and focused on the informational and emotional needs of people and communities'. Some of the supplied messages were models of concise, accurate information: 'Ebola enters your body through your mouth, nose and eyes, or a break in the skin. To catch Ebola you must touch the body fluids of a person with Ebola and then with dirty hands touch your eyes, nose or mouth. Bodily fluids include sweat, stools, vomit, urine, semen, vaginal fluid and blood.' Others were perhaps more dubious: 'Ebola is spread to humans from animals like bats and monkeys. People can catch the disease touching or eating a sick or dead animal,' though it was correctly added 'that now Ebola is in the human population it is being spread from human to human'. But nothing was said about how the informational or emotional needs of the population had been assessed, how empathy was to be acquired, or how specific preventive behaviours were to be promoted.

Instructions predominated: 'Pay your respects [to the dead] without touching, kissing, cleaning or wrapping the body', 'Call the toll free number to arrange [for] the body to be picked up', 'the house, latrine and person's room must be disinfected by trained staff', 'do not care for a sick person at home', and 'soiled clothing and bedding are contagious and must be burnt'. That there would be practical difficulty in responding to these instructions was clear from some of the alternatives then offered. One was to 'contact your local community leader' if the toll-free pick-up call received no answer. Whether the local leader would have any clear idea about what to do, unless specifically trained, remains unsaid.

Another option recognizes that getting a person to a treatment facility might be impractical. In this case, 'if you provide care' (a statement flatly contradicting a previous injunction not to engage in home care), patients were to be isolated in their own space, one person, preferably a survivor, was to be assigned as nurse, and copious liquids were to be provided, in a vessel used only by the patient. Advice was also given on how to improvise protective clothing, with plastic bags to protect the hands, and raincoats worn back to front. But resource constraints are not mentioned, and it is these that determine whether an interesting suggestion becomes an effective technique. Community members might well have asked who would supply the plastic bags and reversible raincoats, or whether the response agency would supply replacements (for burnt clothes and bedding), or what happens if the items are left unattended for a few days to allow the virus to die. Such questions were neither anticipated nor answered.

The document closes with a section on 'what can you do to stop Ebola in your community'. Of six items, three involve speaking with someone to pass the message on, two require the volunteer to educate someone, and one requires contacting a local leader 'to devise ways to inform and engage the community' (more messaging).

This approach to reducing infection expected communities to pass on information and instructions. How well did such an approach work?

Messages, conveyed by radio, poster and loudspeaker van, were received over much of Sierra Leone. This was confirmed by two studies undertaken in late 2014 by Focus 1000.[2] Surveys covered the Freetown area and eleven districts. There was a degree of urban bias, since sampling was weighted towards enumeration areas with larger populations. Village-based surveys in December 2014 showed, however, that the messages had also been clearly received even in remote, off-road, forest-edge villages.

Direct impact of messages on Ebola infections is harder to pin down. Ebola continued to spread and increase in Freetown and surrounding districts in the last three months of 2014, despite intense messaging. At the same time, cases fell in the east and south, in more remote locations where exposure to the main medium, radio, was perhaps rather limited. Kailahun District, the area first experiencing Ebola in Sierra Leone, had its last case on 4 December 2014. It is worth repeating that the epidemic declined first in areas where it first began.

Kailahun District is an especially interesting case, because here there is evidence of decline in infection prior to the major international response. Initial messaging in Kailahun concerned only the risks of forest spillover and bushmeat consumption. At the same time Kailahun provides firm evidence that communities devised effective local responses, including modes of inducing compliance with the demands for behavioural change, once the first shock of the disease had been overcome. This points to a neglected element in Ebola response – the rate at which local learning took place.

Ebola in Jawei chiefdom: a case study in local learning[3]

Kailahun District was the epicentre of the Ebola epidemic in Sierra Leone. Jawei chiefdom, in Kailahun District, had the highest number of Ebola cases in eastern Sierra Leone excepting Nongowa chiefdom, the location for the Kenema ETC, which took patients from all over the country (see Figure 2.5 in Chapter 2).

The first confirmed case of Ebola in Sierra Leone occurred in late May 2014.[4] The victim was a nurse-midwife (MK) working at a community health centre at Koindu, Kissy Teng chiefdom. She had been called to treat a case of Ebola in Guinea, without knowing the risk it posed. The disease arrived in Jawei chiefdom a few days later when Nurse M., trying to reach Kenema hospital, found herself too ill to continue and was admitted to the clinic in Daru.[5] Hearing of her arrival, the wife of the paramount chief hurried to Nurse M.'s bedside, to offer sympathy and help. The two were child-hood friends, born in the same village (Njala Giema, Upper Ngebu section, Jawei chiefdom).

The paramount chief of Jawei chiefdom, Chief Musa Kallon, and other local authorities in Kailahun, were warned by the government about Ebola in March 2014. This was immediately after the Guinea outbreak had been identified as Ebola, but before the disease came to Sierra Leone. This early warning focused on risks of consuming bats and monkeys. But Chief Kallon already had some idea about viral infection risks because he had trained (at Serabu) as a nurse, then as a dispenser, and finally in Freetown as a laboratory technician. He was familiar with Lassa fever, another zoonotic viral disease, which also regularly affects villagers in rural Sierra Leone, and he knew some of the staff of the Lassa fever research unit at Kenema hospital.

On the day in question, however, the chief had been called to Freetown for a meeting. In Freetown, a journalist phoned him to tell him that Ebola had reached Daru. Chief Kallon then called home, to notify his family, and the town chief in Njala Giema, warning of the dangers of touching patients or bodies of Ebola victims. The warning came too late. M. was already dead, and Aminata, the chief's wife, and several staff of the Daru clinic had been infected.

A workshop for health workers was taking place in Daru on the day Nurse M. was admitted to the local hospital. She was a well-known figure in her profession, and many of the participants came to her bedside to sympathize; in all twenty-seven of these visitors became infected and died. The people of Njala Giema failed to heed the chief's warnings about burial, and sixty-eight persons later died in this village as a result of participating in preparation of the corpse.[6]

Chief Kallon tried to get his subjects to suspend normal burial practices, but rumours persisted that Ebola was a political ruse. The chief was known to be a personal friend of the president, and was said to be involved in a plot to reduce opposition votes. Ebola denial was especially strong in Njala Giema, where one of the strongest deniers later died of the disease.

In Freetown, the chief gained permission to leave his meeting early and travel back to Daru. Three days later Aminata herself started to show symptoms. Away that day in Segbwema, a small nearby town, Chief Kallon returned home that evening, and asked for his wife, but she was too ill to come. Chief Kallon insisted she go to Freetown for help, but she died before the journey could be arranged.

The chief decided to put himself in quarantine after he contacted Joseph Bangura of the Tulane University Lassa fever programme, based in Kenema, who told him he suspected it was Ebola. His daughter Jenneh, who had nursed her mother, also became infected and died. Ebola was confirmed and the chief continued a self-imposed quarantine for a total of forty-two days.

At that point Chief Kallon told me he might have become too discouraged to continue, but reminded himself he was descended from warrior stock; 'all is not lost; I go nowhere and fight for the chiefdom I love'. Allowing no one to come physically close to him, he arranged the recruitment and training of fifty-two young men from all parts of the chiefdom, as an anti-Ebola task force. The job of this force was to teach villagers about the disease risks, find the sick, and raise the alarm. It also supplied recruits as surveillance workers, contact tracers and members of burial teams.[7]

Bye-laws were drafted to regulate local movement, and task force members blocked roads. The rule became that if the village chief did not know a visitor that person would be prevented from entering a village. The message was 'no roaming, stay at home'. Even children did not go out to play. Chief Kallon made 'a noise' about Ebola wherever he could, including on the radio, and with agencies such as Médecins sans frontières, who supplied buckets, chlorine and other items.

As the rains were now heavy the chief equipped his force with raincoats and boots. He also paid for his team to go to Kenema, where the virologist, the late Dr Sheik Umar Khan, taught team members how to dress and undress safely using personal protective clothing.[8] People with Ebola were now moving into Daru from outlying districts so local teams sometimes had to bury bodies four or five to a grave. Remarkably, none of the task force volunteers got the virus.[9]

Denial persisted for some time. People avoided Chief Kallon in his compound. On one occasion, a small crowd assembled at his house, on hearing a rumour that his dead wife had appeared to him in a vision. They had hoped to force him to confess that Ebola did not exist. 'But how could they still think Ebola was a plot, since this implied I had killed my own wife?' Task force members were also shunned, and some driven from their homes. The chief housed those who were stigmatized at his compound.

As a result of task force work in identification of cases, contact tracing, movement restrictions and safe burial, infection numbers in Jawi chiefdom began to decline. It was at this point that people began to realize the measures worked, and the rumours began to abate.

The chiefdom experienced 184 Ebola deaths 25 May–28 July 2014, but infection was already ending 'due to the efforts of brave indigenes' (*Awareness Times*, 29 July). Paramount Chief David Keili-Coomber of Mandu called for these local 'best practices' (by-laws, contact tracing and burial teams) 'to be replicated in other parts of the country' (*Awareness Times*, 31 July, see text box, p. 137). The first outside responders wisely attached themselves to these local initiatives.[10] In effect, communities had begun to think like epidemiologists, and epidemiologists (in providing timely and relevant advice to local agents) had begun to think like communities. An evidence-based people's science of Ebola control had begun to emerge.

I asked Chief Kallon what lesson needed to be retained from this experience: his answer was 'learn from earlier mistakes. The denial syndrome was a big problem. We need to learn how to get politics out of Ebola, or similar national emergency responses. People need to understand that some problems affect us all, and are bigger than tribe or party.' He added that the downward curve of the epidemic response reflected growing recognition that the issue was a threat to all – Ebola is a disease, not a party political ruse. But this wisdom should be documented for the future. The story of the Ebola epidemic, he thought, should be taught in every school, so that no Sierra Leonean school child ever forgets.

A further issue he raised was the desirability of continuing the Ebola task force on a permanent basis. Burial ought (he suggested) to become a more sanitary process everywhere, with or without the threat of Ebola. The response teams in Jawei chiefdom were trained by section. Each of eight sections (Sowa, Mano, Kaio, Bobor, Upper Ngebu, Lower Ngebu, Upper Lumegeh, Lower Luengeh) has its own team. (Njala Giema, where so many deaths occurred at the outset, is in Upper Ngebu section.) The team members came from villages in each section. This ensured a social bond between those imposing Ebola control and the people affected by these controls. If local teams were recruited, trained and authorized to carry out 'safe burial' over the longer term, they would do the job 'with respect'.

This would revive an older practice, the chief explained. In former times, young people volunteered to help with burial. The people who did the work of body-washing, carrying of corpses and digging of graves received social recognition in the form of token payments, small gifts, special food, and promotion in the sodalities. Their work was their own 'gift' to the community, in return for blessing. Thus, when there is a funeral, the first to be called out and recognized are the gravediggers and corpse-washers.

With the centrally based burial teams typical of much of the official Ebola response, village people sometimes had to wait four to five days for burial. With locally based teams (organized by chiefdom sections) there would be no delay. The local teams should do everything – the washing, wrapping, grave-digging and so forth. But they struggle for resources – for fuel and transport costs. Chief Kallon also asked that body bags should continue to be supplied, at least until the epidemic was officially declared over. Despite local social acceptance of 'safe burial', those who do the work still tend to be feared and stigmatized, even though none of the volunteers in Jawei had ever been infected. Attention thus needs to be paid to social consequences of stigmatization.

Figure 6.1 Chief Kallon flanked by members of his Ebola task force (Esther Mokuwa seated)

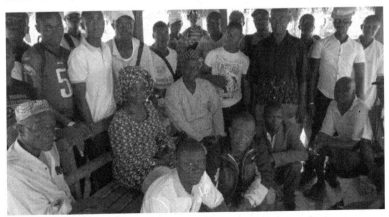

The approach adopted in Jawei chiefdom later became the model for local Ebola response throughout Sierra Leone. Ebola bye-laws were introduced nationally from August 2014, after a conference of chiefs held in the eastern town of Mobai. The security services and other government agencies quickly began to support these local initiatives, so the organizational response resembled that of the army-supported civil defence forces battling the rebel Revolutionary United Front in the civil war in the 1990s. In the south and the east local Ebola task forces were often referred to as 'Ebola kamajoisia' (the name in Mende for special hunters, widely applied during the war to the local civil defence fighters). A more thorough study of task forces, and how they varied in capacity and impact from district to district, is currently under way. Task forces were initially successful at finding cases, reducing inter-village movement and imposing bye-laws. The Jawei force undertook 'safe burial' from the outset, having been trained and equipped before the national Ebola regulations took force. Few agencies were willing initially to build on this example, but later started to recruit and train burial volunteers from chiefdom task forces. Kamajei chiefdom was one instance where burial teams were village-based. Task forces were threatened with marginalization after the militarization of the Ebola response accompanying the international surge from November 2014, but paramount chiefs successfully petitioned State House not to exclude chiefdom task forces from the ramped-up response.

Burial teams (Chief Kallon thought) should also always include women (at least one per team, he suggested). But he admitted to some difficulty in persuading all the women of the chiefdom of his vision for safe and sanitary burial. He noted that he has no power over the Sande women, in matters belonging to their society domain.[11] Techniques of the female body – notably matters relating to childbirth and sexual and reproductive health – remain exclusively under Sande control. This includes the knowledge of procedures to be followed when burying elders of the association. The chief thus acknowledged help from Esther Mokuwa, a member of the UK-based Ebola anthropology response platform,[12] who visited Jawei chiefdom in December 2014 to work with Sande women on 'owning' the Ebola challenge (Figure 6.2).

A Liberian comparison

Sierra Leone was not unique in providing evidence that local responses were important in ending Ebola transmission chains. A case not dissimilar to the one just described has been documented for Lofa County, in north-western Liberia. Like Kailahun District, Lofa County is adjacent to the Ebola epicentre in Guinea, and an early focus for the spread of the disease in Liberia.

In November 2014 the United States Centers for Disease Control sent a team to Lofa County to investigate claims that infection numbers had begun to taper off. The team found evidence the trend was real, and concluded it had been triggered by an unusually effective cooperative relationship between chiefs, communities and international responders.[13]

The first cases of Ebola were reported in Foya, Lofa County, in March, and derived from cross-border infections in Guinea. There were no further cases in April/May, and Liberia hoped it had escaped. But cases began to rise again in June, triggering a more focused response. This included, from the outset, development of a comprehensive response strategy worked out in collaboration with local communities.

The strategy comprised changes in local practices of caring for the sick and burying the dead, the opening of a dedicated ETC in Foya, establishment of a hotline for reporting cases, commissioning of outreach teams, provision of rapid transport and safe burial, establishment of a laboratory for rapid identification, active case-finding, and training of community health volunteers.

Cases rose from twelve in the week ending 14 June to 153 in the week ending 16 August, but declined to only four in the week ending 1 November. This (the authors remark) was the first example in Liberia of a successful strategy to reduce transmission in a country with high cumulative incidence.

The paper describes the creation of an effective environment for communities to come to terms with the disease. The authors note that 'transparency in activities and engagement with the community were central to the response strategy in Lofa'. For example, the Foya ETC was designed without high, opaque walls, to minimize fear of and rumours about what was going on inside. Family members were permitted to visit, either to talk across a fence, or 'inside a ward while wearing full personal protective equipment'. Those who died in the ETC were buried in presence of family members in grave sites marked with clear identification. In the communities, rapid transport of the sick and rapid safe burial 'demonstrated that partners could quickly respond to requests for help'. During safe burials families 'were invited to hold grieving ceremonies according to local customs in memory of the deceased'.[14]

Supervised and unsupervised learning

As noted in Chapter 3, computer engineers distinguish between two processes they refer to as supervised and unsupervised learning,[15] which they apply to different approaches to tuning computational networks based on models of the brain. The distinction can also sometimes be usefully applied to community learning processes.[16]

What has so far been said about community learning in regard to Ebola comprises examples of supervised learning. The international response set parameters for local communities to acquire evidence and draw commonsense conclusions, with Ebola declining as a result of subsequent local behavioural adjustment.

This element of supervision is apparent in an eyewitness account given by Dr Gabriel Rugalema, who led a UN visit to Kenema and

Kailahun districts in the early days of the epidemic.[17] His team arrived in Kailahun town to encounter the District Health Management Committee, security forces and local leaders busy organizing a response, supported by MSF. A recently arrived Canadian mobile field laboratory was about to be assembled. Contact tracing was under way, though hampered by lack of transportation, a situation remedied by the temporary transfer of some FAO vehicles, at Rugalema's request. Likewise, in the Daru case, Chief Kallon, through his medical contacts in Kenema, was in regular receipt of supervisory advice from infectious disease experts associated with the Lassa fever laboratory at Kenema hospital.

In short there was a strong local response to Ebola, but it was underpinned by international assistance. Scope for learning was shaped by these external inputs.

But in some cases a framework to guide the learning process was absent. One instance was the West Point slum in Monrovia. A nervous Liberian government, alarmed at the rapid rise in cases in a post-civil-war urban 'ghetto', settled by a number of ex-combatants, attempted, initially, to close off the area, perhaps mindful of its reputation not just as a slum, but as a home of former fighters.

Ringing West Point with troops created conditions for Ebola to spread further through the ghetto, but also induced some rapid local learning about how to tackle the disease. West Point residents had no other option than to take responsibility for solving a problem with which they had been incarcerated.

After visiting West Point, and then travelling more widely in Liberia and Sierra Leone at the height of the epidemic (November 2014), the journalist Luke Mogelson inferred that self-organized responses to Ebola were widespread in the region:

> Regular West Africans, in the absence of rescue, by the world and by their own governments, which are among the poorest on earth, have proved remarkably adept at finding ways to live and to help others do so. Neighborhoods have mobilized,

health-care workers have volunteered, and rural villagers have formed local Ebola task forces. Individuals who survive Ebola are usually immune to infection, and in many places they have become integral to stemming the epidemic. 'Communities are doing things on their own, with or without our support,' Joel Montgomery, the C.D.C. team leader in Liberia at the time, told me when I met him in Monrovia. 'Death is a strong motivator. When you see your friends and family die, you do something to make a difference.'[18]

The anthropologist Sharon Abramowitz and colleagues[19] provide further evidence that this unsupervised community-driven response was real and effective. They studied fifteen communities in Monrovia and its outskirts in September 2014, via focus groups organized with 386 community leaders, and 'identified strategies being undertaken and recommendations for what a community based response to Ebola should look like'.[20] 'Communities were compelled to generate solutions of their own.'[21]

Leaders were clear about topics such as the need to restrict movement of strangers in and out of communities, the importance of quarantine, and the need to support quarantined households. 'There was a strong community-based ethos informing control measures.'[22] One focus group respondent is quoted as saying 'as a community we keep watch over each other'.

One of the most troublesome issues for practice, however, was a disconnection between messages about not touching, and the practical demands of dealing with a sick person. 'We have heard the messages, but most people do not know how to praticalize them.'[23] The authors of the paper note that caregiving in all its aspects demanded physical contact, but the public health messages regarding physical contact failed to take account of this reality. Some messages said 'don't touch', others said 'touch, but use rubber gloves'.[24]

Faced with this kind of inconsistent advice local opinion moved in its own direction, selecting quarantine as the issue over which communities might have the most meaningful influence. Abramowitz and colleagues sum up the community leader discussions on this topic:

> it was apparent that [leaders] sought to position the community at the centre of the Ebola treatment response by managing the health and safety of quarantined families through food supply, illness surveillance and oversight, reporting, provision of medical supplies, and communication and information.[25]

International responders early on set their face against anything that would smack of 'home care' for Ebola patients, on the grounds that this would multiply the disease. The Monrovia focus groups offered a different perspective. Home care was a moral imperative, especially for women: 'A broad subset of respondents – mainly women – reported that they would care for their sick family members on their own, and that they preferred to do so inside the home.'[26]

So there was a need to think through how home care might be made safer. Focus group members described a plan for isolating themselves with their sick family members and for providing the best locally available appropriate care they could offer, using available resources.

One woman is quoted as saying: 'it will be impossible that my child or husband is sick and I refuse to touch them. I do not have the courage or heart to do that.'[27] Another woman reported that she would find her own protective equipment, 'using a raincoat [and] plastic bags on hands', clearly referencing a widely seen news item regarding Fatu Kekula, the young Liberian nurse who had saved three members of her family, using bin liners for protection (see Chapter 5).[28]

Here, then, was a crucial impasse. A senior international Ebola responder told me bluntly that to advocate 'home care' would be unethical. The Liberian voices referenced by Abramowitz and colleagues imply that to deny the possibility of home care would also be unethical. If international responders resisted moving to support those who refused to abandon what they conceived to be their duty of care then endogenous ways of making home care safe were liable to be pursued.[29] It is apparent that local responses to Ebola embodied an ineradicable element of unsupervised learning.

Changing technique: deliberation or dance?

The Ebola epidemic raised important questions for social science about how behavioural change is achieved. The crisis made apparent a need to return to debates about theories of change.

One approach to change – widely used by agencies working with communities – is based on notions of deliberative decision-making. Participatory rural development draws heavily on the deliberative approach. People meet and explore their problems. They listen to each other. Strategies are proposed. There is debate, disagreement and compromise. Agreements are made to act in various ways. Tasks are allocated, and change is effected.

This is the approach adopted for the community Ebola response in Sierra Leone, based on a set of guidelines for community intervention known as the CLEA Manual (Community Learning for Ebola Action).[30]

The manual states that 'triggering is about stimulating a collective sense of urgency to act in the face of the threat of Ebola, and realize the realities of inaction or inappropriate action'. The natural milieu for deliberation, and for triggering changes in states of mind, is the workshop. The CLEA Manual proposed literally thousands of community workshops.

But there are reasons for wondering whether a deliberative approach – and changes of mind achieved through deliberative interaction – are the most appropriate means through which to approach changes in body technique.

The problem with Ebola is that a natural instinct to care through touching needs to be modified. Deliberation might 'stimulate a collective sense of urgency', but probably through activating conscious checks, including inducing a sense of fear. This might not be the most appropriate way to address the concerns expressed by the Liberian women community leaders quoted by Abramowitz.[31]

As indicated in Chapter 3, Marcel Mauss's seminal paper on techniques of the body initiated a tradition of work on embodiment based on a rather different theory of change – namely, the Durkheimian notion that concepts, categories and mental representations are formed and fixed not through deliberation but through performative action. In particular, the Durkheimians were interested in performative action directed towards sacred ends through which social categories became fixed (or, on occasion, dissolved and formed anew[32]). In short, they were interested in ritual.

The theory of ritual has been mostly used by anthropologists to explain large-scale ceremonial events in 'traditional' society. An instance to which Durkheim himself often alluded was the Australian corroboree. But the approach can be equally well applied to large-scale ceremonial events in any society – for instance, celebration of religious holidays, presidential inaugurations or mourning the war dead. According to Wendy James, the subject of anthropology applies itself root and branch to the study of human beings as ceremonial animals.[33] This explanatory edifice rests on theories of performance. The study of embodiment and movement is freed from asking unhelpful questions such as 'but what does it all mean?' The ceremonial animates. It leads on to the doing of many things, in which deliberation may play little or no part.

A performative approach finds little use for the idea that deliberation triggers a change of mind. In the specific case of Ebola the requirement is to find direct ways of doing (for instance, caring for sick people) that avoid infection risks, but that also avoid hamstringing care through inducing fear and hesitation.

Where, then, can the kinds of performative approaches to behavioural change required to beat Ebola be rehearsed and perfected?

One answer is that the capacity to effect such change already exist in countries like Guinea, Sierra Leone and Liberia, through the performative skills inculcated in rural sodalities such as Poro and Sande. These can be seen as 'workshops' in which dance does the work of deliberation.

The sodalities evolved as a secure and confidential retreat in which small groups could organize around common interests, when beset by many enemies in a dangerous and fluid external world.[34] The sodalities fostered a range of disciplines – from keeping secrets, to enduring pain and hardship, to ways of testing and weeding out spies. Meanings and agreements were danced out by the group, rather than proclaimed or documented.

Expressively, music and dance were thus a major part of the social dynamics of the sodalities. The techniques of the body manifest in dance were major accomplishments expected of both male and female members. An elder who stumbled and missed a beat in a dance might expect to be fined.

Masquerades were both an expression of the sacred values of the society, and a way of publicly expressing the collective power and organization of its members. Society songs sometimes preserved a complex oral record of the linguistically and thus socially mixed origins of its members.

An obvious fact about Ebola was that the super-spreader events were on several occasions the well-attended funerals of society elders. The ritual techniques of the body applied in the burial of these elders are neither known to, nor knowable by, non-members. Nor is it profitable for persons from outside the group to try to know them, since any attempt to penetrate these mysteries is met by group closure.

'Messaging' from non-members about body matters over which the sodalities claim control is wasted effort, since this causes the mechanism of secrecy to snap shut. A logical alternative is to get the members to develop a modified understanding from within.

When Chief Kallon needed to mobilize the women of his chiefdom to support the campaign against Ebola he had to turn to

Figure 6.2 The Daru Sande masquerade, and society elders

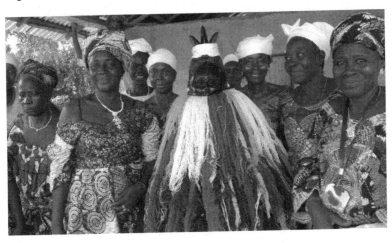

Sande interlocutors to spread the word. He had no power to instruct the women directly. Some were initially opposed to his strategies to cut Ebola infection chains. When I asked him what then happened, he remarked only that the Sande elders went into the bush and danced a solution.

A useful analytical account of the Durkheimian theory of ritual change applied to sodalities in Upper West Africa is provided in the work of the anthropologist Charles Jedrej on Sande ritual dynamics. There he explains that the Mende word *hale* (sometimes translated as 'medicine' but with multiple, apparently disparate meanings) works as a ritual separator. It dissolves old collective understandings, and allows for the reworking of taxonomic elements into new collective representations. According to Jedrej, Sande elders use *hale* as much to adapt to new challenges as to maintain a status quo.[35]

Two Sande elders accompanied Chief Kallon to a workshop at Njala (July 2015) on community mobilization against Ebola and other zoonotic diseases. The visitors from Daru listened patiently to a number of presentations covering deliberative approaches to Ebola control. Eventually, one of the elders asked to speak. Could we help her acquire the white personal protection suit, she asked.

The answer was 'yes' (they cost only $25.00), but we wondered why. She explained that the Sande women had the idea to use the suit to create a dancing 'devil' that would teach the girls of the chiefdom about the Ebola hazard. At times, as Durkheim argued, dance may make more sense than deliberation.

Coda: expressing the need for change

In the Durkheimian tradition of analysis rituals are seen as expressive modes. Ritual action speaks to social circumstances, but does not dictate them. When social circumstances change then so will the rituals expressive of these circumstances. Rituals decay, mutate or erupt as social life demands.

Few in Britain who experienced it will forget the public outpouring of grief that followed the death of Diana, Princess of Wales, in a car crash. The entrance to her London residence was overwhelmed with offerings of flowers. There were so many that the rotting bottom layers of the pile began to cause a public nuisance. Something had to be done. Ritual composers were brought in to create a more suitable venue where public feelings could be vented.

This resulted, eventually, in an imaginative water feature in Hyde Park in which the public could walk barefoot, as somehow seemed appropriate to the memory of someone known as the people's princess. The water feature is constantly on the move, like a stream.

Movement is an almost inescapable feature of most rituals. This is because rituals speak to transitions or renewals. Some take us on a journey. We exit the ritual a different person. Other rituals go round in circles. We begin again with renewed zeal.

Mary Douglas's last book, *Thinking in Circles*, addressed the ancient literary form of poetry constructed as a ring.[36] This was a generalization of her earlier work on the Book of Numbers in the Hebrew Bible,[37] where she had suggested that an allegedly incoherent text was composed as a ring, and for a distinct sociological purpose.

The ancient and fractious tribes were drawn up, in the poem, in marching order, and the ring, decked at strategic points with various items of contested clan history, allowed variant versions to be collated across the ring. The entire ritual structure could be envisaged as rotating through time, carrying its competing claims forward as part of a single entity, like spokes in a wheel.

Whether the poem was ever performed, perhaps as a ring dance, a widespread ancient artistic form expressive of social cohesion, is not known. But given Douglas's description and analysis it is not hard to imagine it might have been.

This brings out one of the objectives that such a ritual performance can attain. By assembling disparate elements into a single experience, apparently contested or contradictory components can be shown to belong to a larger dynamic whole. The overall purpose outweighs troublesome contested or dysfunctional details.

Maybe this approach should have been tried by WHO, when composing its apparently contradictory advice on social mobilization for Ebola: 'home nursing is forbidden' and yet when 'home nursing is unavoidable this is what you should do'. That which is forbidden is attached to the part of the ritual structure speaking of ambulances on paved city streets, and the reversed raincoat is reserved for villages at the end of the forest track. But both belong to the diverse, lively functionality of what people call 'Mama Salong' (Mother Sierra Leone, a ritual being frequently honoured in song and dance, not to mention public exhortations to avoid Ebola risks). A contradiction between home nursing and no home nursing exists only in the straight-line space of a bullet-pointed official release.

A general question arises, 'does ritual composition offer solutions to practical problems'? Could the right kind of composer – poet, dramatist or musician – dynamize the search for safer techniques of the body. The answer is 'yes, perhaps', but only if we first fully understand the social problems to which the ritual must speak. Recall that ritual (and by extension music, poetry and drama) can only speak to underlying social reality; it cannot dictate it.[38]

First we can identify a negative example, an unnecessary performance. Village focus groups sometimes complained that 'we do not even want an ambulance to come to this town, because we hate the crying of an ambulance'.[39] Why did the Ebola ambulance constantly sound its siren, even on remote country roads, where there were no other vehicles to stand aside? If (as information stated) nearly all were bound to die, then please don't cause a noise.

A respectful quietness might have been more appropriate to the deadly reality with which people were coping. Switching off a siren when not absolutely essential may seem a small thing, but it is not a trivial matter to move with quietness and deliberation in the face of death. It shows understanding of local feelings, and from that empathy new patterns of cooperative action and interaction might evolve.

The ritual composer can also inject dynamism where it is sometimes most needed. At times Ebola risked turning emotions from fear to despair, and despair is a very corrosive emotion.

Here is how they do things on the Sierra Leone rice farm, when energy and purpose flag. The purpose of 'ploughing' rice on a Mende upland rice farm is to scatter seed and to dig it in and cover it against birds. This requires rapid 'scratching' with a narrow hoe, to break the crust of the soil and bury the seed, but not too deeply. The task is a major farming bottleneck, since it needs to be done quickly to stop the birds having a feast. The task group is a gang of men, sometimes a pick-up team of brothers or neighbours, but sometimes a regular work gang, supplying labour to its members on a by-turns basis, hoeing in the wake of a skilled broadcaster, with individuals competing to finish stints.

In the 1980s, when I several times took part in such work, a prudent field owner would sometimes also hire a three-man drum band. The Mende slit drum (*kele*) is able to 'talk', and so provides comments on the proceedings, mocking those who are too slow, praising those who do well. To facilitate back-breaking competition members of hoeing groups choose from two styles of hoe, a long-handled and a short-handled. The village blacksmith will generally adjust the handle and pitch of the blade to suit individual arm lengths. Task group members are sometimes as fussy about these adjustments as a concert violinist buying a bow.

Spurred on by the music, the team speeds through the field at accelerated pace. I timed and measured task group stints and found that 20 per cent more ground was covered, on average, when the band was playing than when it was not. But sometimes the women of the farm, who follow on later, to mend patches that have been missed, complain about this high-speed work. In the excitement of the 'dance' the task group has done its work clumsily. The women will also comment if the broadcaster was not up to the mark, throwing too much seed here, and not enough there. But everyone admires that rare breed of expert broadcaster who, for a suitable consideration, will spit rice from the mouth. This truly virtuoso attainment I never even attempted to learn. The result, of course, of all this danced effort is an abundant harvest.

In April 2015, the Kenema singer Ngor Gbetuwa kindly gave me a copy of his Ebola song. I soon discovered he is not the only one to sing about Ebola, and that Ebola-affected Upper West Africa boasts a considerable corpus of music intended to lift spirits and get bodies moving in new and safer ways. Of course, dancing bodies, for the time being, should not touch. There is, in fact, a new dance style, I am told, based on achieving this end – no small feat in crowded events. This encapsulates the argument of this book. If Ebola can so readily evolve its own new dance style, then we should not be surprised if local modifications to techniques of the body have helped end Ebola by spreading as rapidly as the elbow-knock has replaced the handshake as a greeting.

CONCLUSION: STRENGTHENING AN AFRICAN PEOPLE'S SCIENCE

The Upper West African Ebola epidemic of 2013/15 posed an important epistemological question – how does Africa fare when facing a knowledge challenge to which no party has comprehensive solutions in advance.[1] The answer given in this book is that, on the whole, and despite some missed steps, Ebola responders on all levels including the local did surprisingly well in generating necessary new knowledge to beat a terrifying disease.

This book has been an attempt to capture some key aspects of that comprehensive and joint learning process, to ensure a platform can be retained or strengthened for continued readiness and future vigilance. It is striking how rapidly communities learnt to think like epidemiologists, and epidemiologists to think like communities. Local societal capacity to separate categories, and dissolve and reconfigure existing collective representations in response to empirical challenges played an important part.[2]

Thus knowledge has been expanded by the 2014/15 Ebola response, and organized science and West African communities can and ought to continue along a path of co-production of material and social solutions to the threats posed by emergent diseases. Clearly, however, it is a challenge to institutionalize such cooperation, especially given the extreme poverty of many Ebola-affected communities and the intense professionalization of much of medical science.[3]

It is thus worth itemizing some of the main gains of this co-evolved body of knowledge and experience. A first point is to note that the basic approach to control adopted in previous outbreaks in central Africa – isolation of the patient and safe palliative care – also worked at the larger scale of an epidemic involving several countries. The problems of scaling up are challenges of logistics. In particular, the scale and speed of response are crucial – the initial response in Upper West Africa was too slow, and too small in scale; Ebola outbreaks turn into epidemics in regions more densely populated and better provided with roads than the Congo forests.

Secondly, we now know that epidemic models for Ebola need to be recalibrated, to avoid inaccurate projections. This is because risk of infection is non-random in the population as a whole. Those who nurse and bury the sick are at very high risk of infection; those who pass the houses of the sick, even when they live on the same street, have a much lower risk. Abandonment of hand-shaking was probably less a risk reduction strategy than a simple gesture of abstinence signalling public recognition that other, more intimate techniques of the body required to be modified. But the distributed character of West African social intimacy – the network-like features of the extended family – is perhaps not yet fully reflected in epidemiological models.

Thirdly, evidence to suggest that specific sets of social or cultural features influenced the spread of the disease was limited. In the case of gender, infection rates were similar (50:50 for men and women) but the burdens of survival bore down more heavily on women than men. Poor urban neighbourhoods generated a greater-than-average number of high-risk contacts, though in the absence of comparable data for rural areas it is not clear whether this is because of higher levels of extended family networking among more recent migrants to the city. Older people had a greater risk of becoming infected because of their role in nursing and burial. But overall, the disease went as it came, with only limited regard for differences of gender, language, belief, wealth or country. This indicates the importance of general factors in epidemic advance and decline. These might include acquired immunity, but there seems little doubt that the Ebola response itself played a major part.

Fourthly, evidence exists to indicate that some significant part of that effectiveness was a community capacity to respond appropriately to Ebola risks. This was itself based on emergent local knowledge of the disease. The mechanism has been outlined in this book. Ebola-affected populations belonged to moral communities rich in social knowledge, and to those possessing this knowledge, patterns of infection soon became empirically clear. It was readily apparent that corpse-washing or sick-visiting spread the disease, because these were duties indicative of a proper degree of social concern, closely monitored for breaches. People took note if a duty was shirked. This flagged the perverse tendency of the disease to attack those most diligent in carrying out their duties to the sick and dead. Direct empirical inferences were soon drawn about the role of sick-visiting or corpse-washing in sparking further illnesses.

Fifthly, it was learnt (notably by responders such as Médecins sans frontières) that survival rates could be greatly improved by applying palliative treatment, focused on rehydration, to the highest standards possible. Higher survival rates in turn initiated a virtuous cycle of confidence in treatment centres and early reporting. Initial media attention paid to the very high death rates applicable to previous outbreaks of the Zaire species of the Ebola virus was counterproductive because it deterred patients from seeking help. Victims preferred to die at home, where the family would help a transition into the spirit world by guaranteeing a proper burial. Once Ebola came to be seen by responders as not dissimilar to cholera, also a disease which has no cure but which many patients survive through skilled nursing, fear began to dissipate.

Finally, modifications in techniques of the body were central factors in shaping an effective Ebola response, but knowledge had to be generated and applied across communities as well as among medical responders. Emphasis on changing techniques to reduce body contact was crucial in medical response – for example, in the correct design of safe treatment centres to ensure elimination of risks of accidental contact with infected patients. Nursing staff, ambulance crews and burial teams also underwent thorough training in safe donning and removal of protective clothing, and safe ways of treating patients or handling corpses. But less attention was paid to inescapable risks of handling sick and dead bodies at community level, even though these were predictable outcomes of local realities.

Biosafety care protocols for villagers 'waiting for an ambulance' were late additions to the tools of response. Protocols for hammock travel never arrived. 'Safe burial' was introduced not through local consent but through legal sanction. This failed to pay due regard to the social circumstance shaping body technique – that behind every movement, gesture or action lies a rich history of group support and mutually interwoven obligation.

Repeatedly, focus group members asked 'why can't burial teams be recruited and trained locally?' The reason for this request was always the same – that only those socially known to the dead can show proper respect. Some communities demonstrated that they could indeed implement improvised safe nursing and safe burial on their own resources, but turning these demonstrations into an official part of a joined-up Ebola response remains unfinished business. One area where progress is especially needed is in the capacity to determine, quickly, whether burial poses a biosafety risk. Currently, all deaths have to be treated as Ebola deaths where the vast majority pose no threat, for want of rapid and safe field diagnostic kits, capable of being used at the local level.[4]

Something remains to be said about the general problem of how Africa responds to the challenge of science. Science has not always had a good press in Africa. It has often been oversold for reasons more to do with business or political interest. In the past, science was made a legitimation for colonial rule. Today, international corporate interests push science-based solutions to key problems such as African food security. Suspicions are bound to be aroused when science and salesmanship merge. But the fundamental idea of science – that prior judgements must be abandoned in the face of compelling empirical evidence – is of vital significance, if often ill served by development agencies, businesses and governments alike.

What Ebola adds to a more general debate about science in Africa is crucial. This is that, faced with an emergency, rapid empirical adjustments were made, both by communities and by organized science, resulting in the widespread adoption of changes to techniques of the body to reduce infection risk. It is a pattern of discovery to be preserved and developed. One community leader told me he now wanted every child to be taught about Ebola. Making Ebola a central plank for science teaching in schools and colleges might be a fitting and lasting living memorial to those who struggled, suffered and died in the great Upper West African Ebola epidemic of 2013/15.

Let me sum up the message of the book in a few final sentences. Ebola is an emergent disease in Africa. No one knew how to deal with an epidemic, since this was the first epidemic (as opposed to earlier outbreaks). No technical fixes were available; no cures or viable vaccines had yet been developed. Everyone was a learner – responders and communities alike. The evidence suggests that this learning was broadly effective across all three of the worst-affected Upper West African countries – Guinea, Liberia, Sierra Leone – since downturn occurred across the map, and first in the areas where the epidemic first struck. Common elements were experience-based response, and the capacity of external responders to trigger or build on that local response. Where experience of the disease was limited, where the response was disorganized, or where people continued to take risks, perhaps to play politics with the Ebola threat, infection chains persisted.

It will be a long-term remedy if vaccines eventually prove successful, but what the Upper West African epidemic of 2013/15 revealed was an unexpected capacity for communities and responders rapidly to figure out jointly the nature of the infection threat, and then to respond practically in ways that accorded with the evidence. In short, Ebola infection was reduced because people were willing to suspend culture (*pace* Clifford Geertz) long enough to roll out some empirical common sense. The message for future Ebola control seems clear: consolidate ways of working effectively with local communities using basic methods of infection control, and recognize the existence and importance of people's science.

POSTCRIPT

25 February 2016

The Upper West African Ebola epidemic has ended. And so has the international response. The tented Ebola treatment units have been packed. The foreign nurses and doctors have gone. On the outskirts of Bo the gate through which the sick were admitted to the Ebola field hospital swings creaking on the evening breeze, corroded by the chlorine with which it was so often doused. Two of the gatekeepers recreate for us a picture of the facility, and its workings, but only from the footprint left on the ground – a kind of concrete map of what was where. Here was the triage centre; there were the wards. That was where the protective suits were donned; this was where they were removed. The survivors left here; the dead left there. Already the site has become part of the local collective memory, barely eighteen months from when it was built.

So what of the future? No one knows whether the disease will return, or when. The virus lingers in body fluids of survivors and occasional isolated cases are expected from time to time. There may be further epidemics. For now, what remains is the local knowledge gained through coping with a crisis that shook social relations to their core. This knowledge is especially deeply entrenched in the first- and worst-affected communities, which coped largely alone. They are proud, even truculent, about their survival. Quick learning, quick thinking, improvised protection (with plastic bags and the like), and a dogged commitment to the idea of community, shines through their animated accounts. There is also anger that the world should have castigated them for sticking by the sick and dying. Few express a desire for the evident wealth spun off from the international response. Respect for what they did is what they ask.

There may yet be other Ebola epidemics in countries inexperienced in the disease. For sure, there will be other emergent diseases with strong social components to infection. Already the world is seized by a new instance – the spread of Zika virus in the Americas. The general lesson of the Upper West African Ebola epidemic needs to be widely understood, therefore. Common sense, improvisation, distributed practical knowledge and collective action are invaluable elements in a people's science of infection control.

APPENDICES:
EVIDENCE AND TESTIMONY FROM EBOLA-AFFECTED COMMUNITY MEMBERS (CHAPTER 5)

1 Community techniques of burial

1a Male elders: Fogbo

1. The dead body is transferred from the bed to the mat in the room after a *kola* [gift] of Le 1000.00 is given to the husband or wife as a consent to allow those washing the body to set eyes on the nakedness of their partner.
2. 4–6 people [move the body].
3. The dead person is taken from the mat to the backyard for washing. The head is positioned towards the rising of the sun and foot towards the setting of the sun. This is because we believe the spirit of the dead travels to eternity in the direction of the sun. If positioned wrongly, the spirit remains on earth, inflicting pain on family members.
4. In washing, a container or bucket is turned upside down where the feet of the dead person were.
5. The soil from that position [occupied by the bucket] is collected and mixed with some herb (leaves). This mixture is rubbed all over the body of the wife or husband before burial. He or she sleeps with it until the next day [and is then] washed ceremonially. This is done to separate the living from the dead so that the dead will have no power to inflict pain or ill-luck on the remaining members of the family.
6. The dead [person] is taken to church or mosque by 4–5 of his children or close family members. Sorrowful songs are rendered during this part.
7. After prayers, the body is carried to the burial site by 4 to 6 members of the village, while others will be singing songs at the graveside.
8. Dead [person] is placed in the grave and prayer is offered; the pastor or imam throws the first soil on the body in the grave and the second soil is thrown by a family member.

9. In this case it is expected of the last child, that one of the best cloths of the dead [person] is taken to the graveside by a family member (sister or brother) during burial. Part of the soil from the grave is placed on the cloth and placed on the head of the last child. The child then takes this cloth and runs with it to the river or waterside crying. Both the cloth and child are washed in the water. The soil is then thrown into the river indicating the end of a life, as the soil is carried away by the river. The child takes the cloth home and dries it. The cloth belongs to the child and she or he can use it for any purpose they desire.

1b Female elders: Fogbo

1. She was taken by four women, because she's a woman.
2. She was a Christian.
3. Two people removed her cloth from her.
4. Two people washed her; while one was pouring the water, the other was scrubbing her.
5. Yes, she was dressed there by the woman who washed her.
6. Four women took her to the parlour.
7. She has four children, three boys and a girl.
8. Four young men took her to the church for her final prayers.
9. The grave was dug by male youths, I do not know the number because I was not there.
10. She was not buried with [a] casket.
11. Four people (young men) [carried the body to the grave].
12. Two people [prayed], including the pastor.
13. Yes, she was covered with a *lapa* [Krio: wrapper].
14. It was given to the last child; [the wrapper] is drawn from the grave mud, and is placed on the head of the last born of the family, and they will run with to the waterside or stream.
15. The last child after drawing the cloth [*wogu lai*] from the corpse will go to the stream without turning back and the cloth will be placed in the stream. One person [will] accompany him/her and the soaked cloth will be taken to the house and dried under the sun.

1c Youth: Fogbo

1. Family members will gather, decisions are taken, and report is made to chief. Chief approves burial. The body is washed by Muslims or Christians. The body is dressed and the people cry. The body-washing is done by a Christian or Muslim, and sometimes family members. People dig the grave and Muslims conduct burial on Muslims while Christians do the same [for Christians].

2. They pray on the corpse and take the body to the grave site. The grave is overlaid with sticks and grass placed on top of the sticks. Soil is added and the people will offer the final prayer.

2 Treatment of the body in Foindu, a Temne village

How the body is moved from the bed to a mat
The [corpse] is transferred from the bed to a mat in the corner of the room by 4–6 individuals, either family members or elders in the community. While corpse is on the mat, the wife/husband stays by the body to guide [guard?] it.

Washing a corpse requires drainage, at least for Muslims and Christian
The imam or pastor is called to an enclosure in the compound by 4–5 men, for washing; the water used to wash the dead is placed in a hole in an area where people will not step in it so as to avoid the sickness of the corpse spreading in the community.

The body requires to be dressed, and the grave dug
[The] body is dress[ed] with white cloth for Muslims, and for Christians a nice dress of the wife or her husband, [according to] the choice of the children. [The] grave site is prepared by 4–5 young men in community, in the village cemetery.

Appropriate prayers are said for the dead
Family members carry the body to the mosque or church for prayers. If the dead was not praying, the body is prepared in similar manner, except that no pastor/imam will pray on that body; he/she is buried without prayers.

Entombment follows
For Christians and Muslims, when the body is taken to the cemetery, by 4–6 able-bodied men, [the] corpse is placed in the hole by [these] men under the direction of the imam/pastors; prayers are offered at the graveside. Earth is placed on the body by the wife/husband/eldest child/closest family member. With Muslims, sticks and leaves are placed over the dead [body in the grave] before earth/dirt is placed on the body by a very close family member. Water is placed in a bucket outside the house where everyone from the cemetery washes their hands and feet.

Special procedures apply for senior members of the sodalities
In such a case, immediate family member must perform all societal rites before the body can be handed down to them because the dead [body] is [the] legal property of the society. They [the family] also pay redemption fees ([the rate] varies, based on the position in society) before body is taken to the mosque or church.

3 Sodality burial

When a societal head dies, only members of that particular society will be notified, ceremonies are done and the burial ... is completed before pronouncing the death. Only those who belong to the society go to the grave site. An invisible [masked?] devil will carry the corpse to the grave. After all the burial practices, the invisible devils will start appearing, [but] only members will stay outside, non-members lock themselves in [their] rooms. (Town chief, Gbo chiefdom)

The death of the chief is not pronounced immediately. The corpse is taken to the mortuary. The consent of the paramount chief of that chiefdom and other chiefs is sought. Later the death pronouncement is made to the family and town. (Section chief)

Firstly, nobody will announce the death without permission. The chiefs will meet at a secret location and arrange all that needs to be done (ceremonies). The body will be buried at a special place and a masked devil does the burial in some chiefdoms. (Town crier, Baiima, Gbo chiefdom)

If a man, ceremonies are observed before the family members will be asked to collect the corpse for burial. In some instances the corpse will be buried in a sacred bush. The same is done for women. (Farmer, Gbo chiefdom)

The corpse is never buried in the day, but during the night due to customs and traditions. (Farmer, Mokebe, Gbo chiefdom)

When a societal head dies, no one is to cry until it is declared by the societal head. [People] will be told that the person is in a state of unconsciousness. All the societal heads will converge in the village. A thin thread is passed around the house to prevent non-members entering [to see] the body. When all have converged, the chief will report that the societal head is in a state of coma. And they will start to dance and sing. A fine is levied on the family. When they pay, the society people will declare that their head is dead. The society people will perform their ceremony and hand over the body to the chief, who in turn will give [it to] the family. The religious [people] are called to pray on the corpse, thereafter the body is returned to the societal head and it will be buried in a secret location. The fine levied on the family is [for the amount] he or she has been eating. Now that [the societal head] is dead s/he should refund all to the society members before permission is granted for the burial. (Women elders, Sanola Gaura)

4a Disquiet at burial team actions in a Mende village (Baiima)

I am not happy at all because our relatives are not included in the burial process.

I am not happy because the dead are not washed and not buried properly as required by us. Even the chemical they use on dead bodies is not required.

I am not happy because [the dead] are not properly buried (not well covered).

The Ebola burial team is supposed to include people in our community as well. The bodies of the dead are supposed to be wash[ed] and prayers are offered.

Let our people be trained as contact tracers, [and] burial team [members], and [let them] offer or be allowed to work in the Ebola team, so we can handle the disease properly.

Train communities to be burying their dead, and to give all materials to the community for safe burial practices.

4b Disquiet at burial team actions in a Temne village (Foindu)

No, we are not pleased with the manner in which the burial team treats our dead relative.

Dead are buried without clothes (clean decent cloth). Family members in most cases do not witness the death of their loved ones [because they die in a distant care centre].

No form of religious prayer was offered. Burial teams are all men, burying both men and women.

Dead bodies are dumped into the grave without care and respect.

Cultural issues are neglected.

The grave is not sufficiently covered.

[We want] that government trains burial team at chiefdom level, so that they will honour and respect the dead.

We are willing to be trained, and equipped to do the work with care. Tribal and regional differences should be taken into account.

5a Experiences with Ebola quarantine

The village was quarantined for 21 days and World Food Programme provided food during the quarantine. (Bawuya, Kori, female elders)

Houses and homes were isolated with sick people before they were transported to holding centres. The sick were cared for by brothers and sisters around them; Ebola persons were sent to Moyamba treatment centre. (Moyamba Junction, youths)

House is closed and flagged with red tape. None is allowed to enter the house until the body is buried and the house sanitized for 3 days. (Moyamba Junction, youths)

Yes, we are no longer working, and people are not doing things to keep life moving. No business, and we last received supply on the 3rd and 21st [October]. We have not received for the past 3 months. (Moyamba Junction, male elders)

During the 21 days [quarantine] we had supply from WFP [World Food Programme]; since then no other help. We are very poor. Red Cross also registered us but has not given supply since. (Moyamba Junction, male elders)

The entire village was quarantined for 21 days. The town was full with soldiers and police. The village was quarantined two times. WFP provided rice, oil, beans and salt, during our first quarantine without security. (Fogbo, Kori, women elders)

5b Historical experiences with quarantine for other sicknesses

[Smallpox] Affected people were taken to a separate place for medication (Mogbisi, Gbo, male elders' group)

[Smallpox] We were not allowed to mingle with our companions until we became better. (Mokebe, Gbo, female elders' group)

[Measles?] Isolation to a bush in the daytime to prevent spread and return to home at night. (Moyamba Junction, Fakuniya)

[Measles] Isolation in daytime – in an old farmhouse. Now controlled by vaccination. (Fogbo, Kori, youth group)

5c Goat Plague [PPR]: a model for Ebola?

[symptoms are] watery stool from goats, bloating stomach and tears run from their eyes, water runs from their mouth. Four goats [were] infected. Infected goats are taken to different locations ([to be in] isolation [= quarantine]). (Mogbisi, Gbo, male elders' group)

[symptoms are] mucus excretion, diarrhoea, hair loss. In 2013 over 50 goats died; all died and that stopped the spread. (Fogbo, Kori, youth group)

[Action needed] To bury the affected [animal]. Remove all affected ones from the nonaffected. (Mokebe, Gbo, female elders' group)

[Impact, action needed] Over 40 [animals were infected]. The affected ones should be removed from the non-affected. (Fengehun, Kakua, male elders' group)

[Impact, action needed] Nearly all died. Prevent other animals from coming in contact with infected animal. (Fengehun, Kakua, youth group)

6 Village questions about Ebola

Bo-Gaura

[Is there] any plan of assisting us with some medicine for the treatment of common sicknesses like malaria?

How can [we] go [to hospital] with the sick when there is no motorbike or road?

It has been said [in] bye-laws that we should not touch dead bodies; what can we do if somebody [has] died, considering the distance?

Why did the authorities delay in intervening to stop the spread of this deadly disease?

Treat all sicknesses including malaria [not just Ebola].

Jagbema-Gaura

Why is it that [the] government has mounted checkpoints with security personnel as a means to cure Ebola?

Where is all the money sent by the West, and donors, going?

Our people are still dying.

Government should create a facility for village people to get basic training on health issues and [be] given some incentives.

Why are infected corpses buried in other towns rather than in their home towns. Government should establish a health centre close to us in the village.

Njala-Gaura

Since the symptoms of Ebola are fever, headache, joint pain, etc., do we take for granted that anybody with those symptoms has Ebola?

We always hear from people [about] huge amounts to Sierra Leone to stop this Ebola, but yet people are dying, why?

Senehun Buima-Gaura

People say there is no treatment for Ebola, [so] why do they ask people to go for treatment?

They say there is no medicine for Ebola, [so] how are they treating people with the sickness if there is no medicine?

NOTES

Introduction

1   Properly Ebola Virus Disease, or EVD. I will continue to use the short form. Ebola is the name of a river in the Democratic Republic of Congo, and it was chosen to avoid the risk of stigmatizing the small town, 60 kilometres distant, where the first known outbreak occurred (*BBC News Magazine*, 18 July 2014).

2   www.ibtimes.co.uk/ebola-discoverer-peter-piot-i-would-sit-next-infected-person-tube-1459154, 31 July 2014.

3   A second countdown was completed on 17 March 2016, the day a further case cluster was reported in Guinea.

4   Douglas (1992).

5   I owe the phrase to Daniel B. Cohen.

6   Mauss (1973 [1935]).

7   Durkheim (1995 [1912]).

8   Schlanger (2006).

9   There is better news on vaccines. One vaccine candidate has been shown to be promisingly effective (Henao-Restrepo et al. 2015) when deployed via 'ring vaccination' to protect those with high exposure to the disease (mainly family carers and medical responders).

10   Hobart (1993).

11   The archaism was probably deliberate. Upper Volta (the former name for Burkina Faso) was a stand-in for any remote part of Africa of little conceivable interest to the UK government.

12   Dant (2005).

13   Richards (1985).

14   O'Carroll (2015).

1   The world's first Ebola epidemic

1   Hewlett and Hewlett (2008).

2   Richards et al. (2015).

3   Weber (1930), Tawney (1977 [1926]).

4   Durkheim (1995 [1912]).

5   For example Karan and Pogge (2015).

6   As offered by the neo-Durkheimian sociologist Randall Collins (2004).

7   Oosterhoff et al. (2015).

8   Fallah et al. (2015).

9   On the other hand, the less densely populated peri-urban fringes of the three capital cities proved to be rather fertile terrain for Ebola spread. Numbers of cases were significantly higher per head of population in peri-urban Freetown than in the inner-city slums, for example (author's unpublished data).

10   See the section on literature in the entry for Ebola Virus Disease in Wikipedia (en.wikipedia.org/wiki/Ebola_virus_disease#Literature).

11   Patent US 20120251502 A1, 'Human Ebola virus species and compositions and methods thereof", filing date: 26 October 2009.

12   As alleged in a report in the Iraqi newspaper *al Sabaah* ('Daash Ebola transferred to Mosul', 31 December 2014), citing an unnamed source.

13   www.who.int/csr/disease/ebola/overview-august-2014/en/.

14   Kamins et al. (2011).

15   Recent work in Sierra Leone establishes that bat eating is quite common in some communities (personal communication, Roland Suluku).

16   One of these stories comes from villagers on the Guinea border in Kissy Teng, who speak of an earlier case of a woman who showed Ebola-like symptoms and later recovered (fieldwork, March 2016).

17   Gire et al. (2014).

18   Park et al. (2015).

19   Ibid., p. 1518.

20   Ibid.

21   As remarked by Bob Geldof.

22   Stadler et al. (2014).

23   Maxmen (2015).

2   The epidemic's rise and decline

1   Lovejoy (2005: 95).

2   Fairhead et al. (2003).

3   A system of indirect rule (rule through indigenous institutions) modelled on that prevailing in the protectorate of Sierra Leone was adopted by Liberia at the end of the first decade of the twentieth century as a framework for more effective administration of interior districts.

4   For one account see 'Womey massacre' at en.wikipedia.org/wiki/Womey_Massacre.

5   Baize et al. (2014).

6   Focus 1000 (2014a, 2014b).

7   Richards et al. (2015), questionnaire responses, survey data sets, December 2014.

8   The first Ebola cases in Sierra Leone emerged (in March 2014) in two villages

close to a crossing point on the Moa river at Nongowa, a small Guinean town important in the regional trade in kola nuts.

9 When I visited Sandeyalu (Kissi Kama chiefdom) in 2002, shortly after the end of the civil war in Sierra Leone, schoolchildren in the village greeted me in French. English and Krio were languages they associated with their older siblings. Hitherto, they had known only refugee life in Guinea.

10 Alldridge (1901: 215).

11 Not to be confused with Koidu, the commercial centre of the diamond district of Kono.

12 *Hoku = Aku* (we greet), the name by which (Nigerian) Yoruba people are often known in Sierra Leone. *Lapa* derives from Dutch (*lappen* – pieces [of cloth]). This is presumably a linguistic relic of Dutch cloth traders based at Cape Mount in the mid-seventeenth century.

13 The town was hugely damaged during the war, and even today is but a shadow of its former self. Many Guinea traders abandoned their large houses in Koindu and relocated to the Guinean side of the border. This helps account for the large recent rise in the population of Gueckedou.

14 Currently, the road reaches Pendembu, about twenty-five kilometres from Kailahun.

15 Villagers interviewed in Kisi Teng chiefdom in March 2016 claimed the first case of Ebola (in Sokuma) pre-dated the reported origin of the epidemic in Guinea in December 2013. This suggests that more remains to be discovered about the origins of the epidemic than has so far been reported. But there seems little doubt that cross-border networking, by Kissi villagers, by Mandingo and Fula traders, and by local medical practitioners, played a significant part in the early spread.

16 Interview with paramount chief of Jawei chiefdom, May 2015 (see Chapter 6).

17 Ibid.

18 Henao-Restrepo et al. (2015).

19 www.who.int/csr/disease/ebola/situation-reports/en/.

20 Hewlett and Hewlett (2008).

21 Ministry of Social Welfare et al. (2014).

22 Abramowitz et al. (2015).

23 Mogelson (2015).

24 O'Carroll (2015).

25 CDC (2014).

26 MSF, Liberia, 20 January 2015, Sierra Leone, 24 January 2015.

27 Scarpino et al. (2014); see also Weitz and Dushoff (2015).

28 Richards et al. (2015).

29 Fithen and Richards (2005).

3 Washing the dead

1   *The Australian*, 6 November 2014.
2   Interview by Associated Press, 4 December 2014.
3   'Dumped like an animal': Women's focus group, Fengehun, Kakua, December 2014.
4   The interested reader is referred to the excellent analysis by Kuper (1998).
5   Geertz (1983).
6   Durkheim (1995 [1912]).
7   Ibid., p. 218.
8   Berger and Turow (2011).
9   Kuper (1998); Douglas (2004).
10 Durkheim and Mauss (1963 [1902/03]).
11 Mauss (1973 [1935]).
12 And how is the bucket carried?; see Van der Niet (2009).
13 Richards et al. (2015).
14 Women elders, Peri-Fefewabu, Gaura chiefdom, Kenema District, a village with direct experience of Ebola cases, December 2014.
15 From the field report of Fomba Kanneh, Bo-Gaura, Kenema District, December 2014.
16 Picton (2000).
17 Nuijten et al. (2009).
18 Nuijten and Richards (2011).
19 Mokuwa (2015).
20 These voices (to be analysed below) were eventually heard via the Ebola Response Anthropology website. Some later burial teams were then recruited and trained locally. An example is the burial team in Kamajei chiefdom, trained in a nearby chiefdom headquarters, Mano (interview with the town chief, Mamawa Tarawali, in Mogbuama, Kamajei chiefdom, 27 March 2016).

4 Ebola in rural Sierra Leone

1   Sterne (2003).
2   McFeat (1972); Brooks (1995 [1975]).
3   Douglas (1986).
4   Gustav Holst, *Seven Parts Songs for Female Voice, Chorus and Strings*, Op. 44.
5   Cumulative confirmed Ebola cases in Sierra Leone at 24 December 2015 were 8,704. About half of these were recorded in urban areas.
6   Richards (1986).
7   Summaries of questionnaire responses and transcripts of focus group sessions are available in the form of appendices to eight reports written for the Social Mobilization Action Consortium (SMAC) funded by UK Aid, and posted to

the Ebola Response Anthropology Platform website (www.ebola-anthro
pology.net).

8   Gender does not appear to be a significant variable in explaining variations in
responses to these two questions.

9   The differences between the answers to the two questions are statistically
significant at the 95 per cent confidence level.

10   Senehum-Buima, a forest-edge village in Gaura chiefdom, December 2014.

11   The difference is statistically significant, according to the Fisher exact test, at
the 95 per cent confidence level.

12   Richards et al. (2015).

13   Oosterhoff et al. (2015).

14   Numbers were sometimes lower in smaller villages, where all available adults
were interviewed.

15   There was one missing answer.

16   Bo-Gaura, all groups.

17   Bawuya, female youth.

18   Peri Fefewabu, various youths.

19   Bawuya, female youth leader.

20   Richards (1986).

5   Burial technique

1   Bawuya, Kori, youth group. A similar practice – the 'washing' of widows – is
described in detail in Ferme (2001) for a Mende village in Wunde chiefdom.

2   WHO (2014b).

3   Foindu, Yoni, youth group.

4   Ibid.

5   Male elders, Bo-Gaura, Gola forest.

6   Mogbuama, Kamajei.

7   Moyamba Junction, youths.

8   Peri Fefewabu, youth group.

9   Mobai, Kamajei, male elders.

10   Bo, December 2014.

11   Male, age twenty-one, Bo, December 2014.

12   I owe the notion of the 'invention of ignorance' to the title of a book by Mark
Hobart (1993).

13   WHO (2014b).

14   Parsons (1997).

15   Ibid., Abstract.

16   For example: 'The Ebola outbreak in West Africa has claimed the lives of over
9000 people largely due to a combination of poor health care infrastructure
in affected countries, traditional beliefs and cultural practices, including

the consumption of bushmeat and certain burial rituals that have amplified transmission' (Karan and Pogge 2015).

17 But on occasion, Ebola survivors did speak about harassment: 'they ... come with guns to threaten us, and when you are diagnosed to have Ebola, they arrest you. That alone makes you to be depressed, and not for the disease but [because] of the forces surrounding [you]. The entire family [is] looked at negatively.' (Ebola survivor, interviewed in Bo town, December 2014.)

18 Several times I heard the comment that the slow process of ending Ebola infection pathways in Sierra Leone owed something to local political in-fighting.

19 Ebola survivor, female, age thirty, Bo, December 2014.

20 Ebola survivor, female, age twenty, Bo, December 2014, younger sister of the person cited above.

21 Lamontagne et al. (2014).

22 Hewlett and Hewlett (2008).

23 Cohen (2014).

24 Foindu, Yoni, Tonkolili District, youth group, December 2014.

6 Community responses to Ebola

1 Geertz (1983).

2 Focus 1000 (2014a, 2014b).

3 The account was given to the author by Paramount Chief Musa Ngombuka Kallon II, of Jawei chiefdom, in an interview in Daru on 22 May 2015.

4 Enquiries (March 2016) in Kpondu, a village in Kissy Teng chiefdom, close to the Guinea border, suggests this may have been the first place in Sierra Leone with an Ebola outbreak. People here date the first case to March 2014. The village schoolteacher compiled a record as events unfolded, and recorded over twenty cases up until August 2014, after which there were no further cases. A young man who survived the disease told us he was taken to the ETC in Gueckedou (Gegedu) in Guinea because the facility in Kailahun had not yet been built.

5 The date in my field notes is 25 May 2014, but it is not clear whether this was the date on which Nurse M. travelled to Daru or the date she first became ill. An article by Abdul R. Thomas, in the *Sierra Leone Telegraph*, 28 May 2014, cites a radio interview by Brima Kargbo (government Chief Medical Officer) as stating that 'Three people of the same family have died of the deadly Ebola virus in Sokoma village, Kissy Teng chiefdom. The first victim was a female herbalist who has frequently been travelling to Guinea. The herbalist died three weeks ago ... The Ministry of Health was informed on 22nd May' ... Seven other suspected cases were also reported, after they had attended funerals. Nurse M. appears to have been infected when these subsequent

cases were brought to the Koindu Community Health Centre. Sokoma is the neighbouring village to Kpondu. Villagers in Kpondu claimed their own village was first infected.

6   The Njala-Giema case is currently being followed up by an Njala research team. We were told (23 February 2016) that there were eighty-nine Ebola cases in all (twenty-one survivors) in a period beginning in early June 2014. Located on the road from Daru to Joru skirting the northern margins of the Gola forest, Njala Giema is a typical compact, medium-sized, somewhat isolated Mende forest-edge village. Transporters found ways to bypass the village, which ran short of salt as a result. Ebola cases represented between a quarter to a third of all adults. Every residential quarter had infections. It seems probable most adults were high-risk contacts. Infection transmission may have been ended by isolation and quarantine, perhaps combined with some element of acquired immunity (O'Carroll 2015).

7   This was before emergency legislation required all burial to be carried out by official burial teams.

8   Dr Sheik Umar Khan was the country's leading Lassa fever specialist. Later he too caught Ebola, and died on 29 July 2014, a shattering and demoralizing loss, felt throughout the country and internationally.

9   Interview by the author with task force members, Daru, 20 October 2015.

10   See 'How Kailahun District kicked Ebola out', WHO December 2014, www.who.int/features/2014/kailahun-beats-ebola/en/.

11   Jedrej (1974, 1976a, 1976b).

12   www.ebola-anthropology.net.

13   Sharma et al. (2014).

14   A similar positive response to makeshift community treatment centres in Sierra Leone is reported by Oosterhoff et al. (2015). These were intended as temporary holding centres, but owing to the rise in the number of cases became alternatives to more distant ETCs, and were staffed by local workers, not all of whom were medically trained. But with workers recruited locally families could easily get information about a patient's progress, and even at times see or talk to loved ones through the open-sided tents. This reduced fear of the disease and stemmed rumours about the hidden purposes of distant ETCs (e.g. fear of organ harvesting).

15   Picton (2000).

16   Richards et al. (2009).

17   30 June and 1 July 2014.

18   Mogelson (2015).

19   Abramowitz et al. (2015).

20   Ibid., p. 1.

21   Ibid., p. 3.

22   Ibid., p. 8.

23 Ibid.

24 Ibid., p. 9.

25 Ibid., p. 11.

26 Ibid.

27 Ibid.

28 Reported by CNN at http://edition.cnn.com/2014/09/25/health/ebola-fatu-family/index.html.

29 CLEA (2014) Community-Led Ebola Action field guide for community mobilisers, Freetown, Community Mobilization Action Consortium (SMAC), GOAL and Restless Development.

30 This point is now explicitly recognized in a very interesting discussion of ethical challenges raised by the West African Ebola epidemic by Calain and Poncin (2015).

31 Abramowitz et al. (2015).

32 Richards (2015).

33 James (2003).

34 A celebrated paper by the German sociologist Georg Simmel (1906) first proposed that secret societies, as a sociological phenomenon, were an organizational reaction to conditions of high external insecurity. Although Simmel's paper is lacking in ethnographic detail, he mentions the existence of African secret societies, and may have had some knowledge of Poro and Sande from the well-informed descriptions of these sodalities in a book on Western Liberia by the Swiss zoologist Buettikofer, published in German in the 1890s (Richards 2015).

35 Richards (2015).

36 Douglas (2007).

37 Douglas (1993).

38 However, it is worth adding that dancing can offer a number of important back channels for communication. See, for example, Adam Zamoyski's entertaining account of the dances and social occasions attached to the Congress of Vienna, where the post-Napoleonic future of Europe was negotiated, through which a number of informal diplomatic understandings were facilitated (Zamoyski 2001).

39 Mogbuama, Kamajei, women's focus group.

Conclusion

1 This book thus differs from my earlier *Indigenous Agricultural Revolution* (Richards 1985), where crop selection by African farmers was shown to out-compete international crop science in local conditions. In this earlier case, both parties were rich in prior knowledge. The present case is one in which both parties started from positions of considerable ignorance.

2   Richards (2015).

3   Some of these issues are addressed in an important assessment of lessons
     learned from Ebola, Moon et al. (2015). This report flags but does not elaborate
     on the importance of community response.

4   All three countries had completed the time period without cases for the region
     to be declared free of Ebola by 17 March 2016, the day on which a new case
     cluster emerged in southern Guinea traced to lingering infection in a survivor.
     Three new cases in Liberia were also linked to this outbreak. Rapid containment
     measures have been put in place, including ring vaccination among high-risk
     contacts. Other similar isolated cases are expected to emerge, probably mainly
     through sexual transmission, and these could ignite new infection chains where
     (as appears to have been the case just mentioned) 'safe burial' was neglected.

REFERENCES

Abramowitz, S. A. et al. (2015) 'Community-centered responses to Ebola in urban Liberia: the view from below', *PLOS Neglected Tropical Diseases*, 9 April, doi: 10.1371/journal.pntd.0003706.

Alldridge, T. (1901) *The Sherbro and Its Hinterland*, London: Macmillan.

Baize, S. et al. (2014) 'Emergence of Zaire Ebola Virus Disease in Guinea – preliminary report', *N. Engl. J. Med.*, 16 April, PubMed PMID: 24738640.

Bausch, D. G. and L. Schwarz (2014) 'Outbreak of Ebola Virus Disease in Guinea: where ecology meets economy', *PLoS Negl. Trop. Dis.*, 8(7): e3056, doi: 10.1371/journal.pntd.0003056.

Berger, J. and G. Turow (eds) (2011) *Music, Science and the Rhythmic Brain: Cultural and clinical implications*, New York and London: Routledge.

Brooks, F. (1995 [1975]) *The Mythical Man-month*, Addison-Wesley.

Calain, P. and M. Poncin (2015) 'Reaching out to Ebola victims: coercion, persuasion or an appeal for self-sacrifice?', *Social Science and Medicine*, 147: 126–33, dx.doi.org/10.1016/j.socsciemed.2015.10.063.

CDC (Centers for Disease Control and Prevention) (2014) 'Estimating the future numbers of cases in the Ebola epidemic – Liberia and Sierra Leone, 2014–2015', *MMWR (Mortality and Morbidity Weekly Report)*, 26 September.

CLEA (2014) Community-Led Ebola Action field guide for community mobilisers, Freetown, Community Mobilization Action Consortium (SMAC), GOAL and Restless Development.

Cohen, E. (2014) 'Woman saves three relatives from Ebola', *CNN News*, 26 September.

Collins, R (2004) *Interaction Ritual Chains*, Princeton, NJ: Princeton University Press.

Dant, T. (2005) *Materiality and Society*, Maidenhead: Open University Press.

Douglas, Mary (1986) *How Institutions Think*, London: Routledge and Kegan Paul.

—— (1992) *Risk and Blame: Essays in cultural theory*, London: Routledge.

—— (1993) *In the Wilderness: The doctrine of defilement in the book of Numbers*, Oxford: Oxford University Press.

—— (2004) 'Traditional culture: let's hear no more about it', in V. Rao and M. Walton (eds), *Culture and Public Action*, Stanford, CA: Stanford University Press, pp. 85–108.

—— (2007) *Thinking in Circles: An essay on ring composition*, New Haven, CT, and London: Yale University Press.

Durkheim, É. (1995 [1912]) *Elementary Forms of Religious Life*, trans. K. Fields, New York: Free Press.

Durkheim, É. and M. Mauss (1963 [1902/03]) *Primitive Classification*, trans. R. Needham, Chicago, IL: University of Chicago Press.

Fairhead, J. et al. (2003) *African-American Exploration in West Africa: Four nineteenth century diaries*, Bloomington: Indiana University Press.

Fallah, M., L. Skrip, S. Gertler, D. Yamin and A. Galvani (2015) 'Quantifying poverty as a driver of Ebola transmission', *PLOS Neglected Tropical Disease*, 31 December 31, doi: 10.1371/journal.pntd.0004260.

Ferme, M. C. (2001) *The Underneath of Things: Violence, history and the everyday in Sierra Leone*, Berkeley: University of California Press.

Fithen, C. and P. Richards (2005) 'Making war, crafting peace: militia solidarities and demobilization in Sierra Leone', in P. Richards (ed.), *No Peace, No War: Learning to live with violent conflict*, Oxford: James Currey, pp. 117–36.

Focus 1000 (2014a) 'Study on public knowledge, attitudes, and practices relating to Ebola Virus Disease (EVD) prevention and medical care in Sierra Leone', Report KAP-1, September, Freetown, Sierra Leone.

—— (2014b) 'Follow-up study on public knowledge, attitudes, and practices relating to Ebola Virus Disease (EVD) prevention and medical care in Sierra Leone', Report KAP-2, December, Freetown, Sierra Leone.

Geertz, C. (1983) 'Common sense as a cultural system', in *Local Knowledge: Further essays in interpretive anthropology*, New York: Basic Books, pp. 73–93.

Gire, S. K. et al. (2014) 'Genomic surveillance elucidates Ebola virus origin and transmission during the 2014 outbreak', *Science*, 28 August.

Henao-Restrepo, A. M. et al. (2015) 'Efficacy and effectiveness of an rVSV-vectored vaccine expressing Ebola surface glycoprotein: interim results from the Guinea ring vaccination cluster-randomised trial', *Lancet*, 386(9996): 857–66, published online 3 August.

Hewlett, B. S. and B. L. Hewlett (2008) *Ebola, Culture and Politics: The anthropology of an emerging disease*, Belmont, CA: Thomson Wadsworth.

Hobart, M. (ed.) (1993) *An Anthropological Critique of Development: The growth of ignorance*, London: Routledge.

James, W. (2003) *The Ceremonial Animal: A new portrait of anthropology*, Oxford: Oxford University Press.

Jedrej, C. (1974) 'An analytical note on the land and spirits of the Sewa Mende', *Africa: Journal of the International African Institute*, 44(1): 38–45.

—— (1976a) 'Structural aspects of a West African secret society', *Journal of Anthropological Research*, 32(3): 234–45.

—— (1976b) 'Medicine, fetish and secret society in a West African culture', *Africa: Journal of the International African Institute*, 46(3): 247–57.

Kamins, A. et al. (2011) 'Uncovering the fruit bat bushmeat commodity chain and the true extent of fruit bat hunting in Ghana, West Africa', *Biological Conservation*, 144(12): 3000–8, doi: 10.1016/j.biocon 2011.09.003.

Karan, A. and T. Pogge (2015) 'Ebola and the need for restructuring pharmaceutical incentives', *J. Glob. Health*, published online 11 February, doi: 10.7189/jogh.05.010303.

Kuper, A. (1998) *Culture: The anthropologists' account*, Cambridge, MA, and London: Harvard University Press.

Lamontagne, F., C. Clément, T. Fletcher, S. T. Jacob, W. A. Fischer II and R. A. Fowler (2014) 'Doing today's work superbly well: treating Ebola with current tools', *New England Journal of Medicine*, 24 September, updated 25 September, NEJM.org., doi: 10.1056/NEJMp1411310.

Lovejoy, P. (2005) 'Kola in the history of West Africa', in *Ecology and Ethnography of Muslim Trade in West Africa*, ch. 4, Trenton, NJ, and Asmara, Eritrea: Africa World Press, pp. 87–127.

Mauss, M. (1973 [1935]) 'Les techniques du corps', *Journal de psychologie*, 32: 271–93, trans. B. Brewster and published as 'Techniques of the body' in *Economy and Society*, 2(1): 70–88, 1973.

McFeat, T. (1972) *Task Group Cultures*, Oxford: Pergamon.

Ministry of Social Welfare, Gender and Children's Affairs, UN Women, Statistics Sierra Leone and Oxfam (2014) *Report of the multi-sector impact assessment of gender dimensions of the Ebola Virus Disease (EVD) in Sierra Leone*, Freetown, 31 December.

Mogelson, L. (2015) 'When the fever breaks', Letter from West Africa, *New Yorker*, 19 January.

Mokuwa, A. (2015) 'Management of rice seed during insurgency: a case study of Sierra Leone', PhD thesis, Wageningen University, Netherlands.

Mokuwa, E. Y. (2014) 'Speaking truth to power? Using the focus group to make a qualitative assessment of a field experiment in rural development, Report to the International Initiative on Impact Evaluation (3IE), revised after peer review in August 2014; to be submitted for publication.

Moon, S. et al. (2015) 'Will Ebola change the game? Ten essential reforms before the next pandemic. The report of the Harvard-LSHTM independent panel on the global response to Ebola', *Lancet*, 22 November, dx.doi.org/10/1016/50140-6736(15)00946-0.

Nuijten, E. and P. Richards (2011) 'Pollen flows within and between rice and millet fields in relation to farmer variety development in The Gambia', *Plant Genetic Resources: Characterization and Utilization*, doi: 10.1017/51499262111000048I.

Nuijten, E., R. van Treuren, P. C. Struik, A. Mokuwa, F. Okry, B. Teeken and P. Richards (2009) 'Evidence for the emergence of new rice types of interspecific hybrid origin in West-African farmer fields', *PLOS ONE*, 4(10), 6 October.

O'Carroll, L. (2015) 'Ebola study finds women in Guinea who appear immune to the virus', *Guardian*, 15 October.

Oosterhoff, P., E. Y. Mokuwa and A. Wilkinson (2015) *Community-based Ebola Care Centres: A formative evaluation*, Ebola Response Anthropology Platform, London School of Hygiene and Tropical Medicine and Institute of Development Studies at the University of Sussex.

Park, D. J. et al. (2015) 'Ebola virus epidemiology, transmission, and evolution during seven months in Sierra Leone', *Cell*, 161: 1516–26, 18 June.

Parsons, B. (1997) 'Change and development in the British funeral industry during the 20th century, with special reference to the period 1960–1994', PhD thesis, University of Westminster.

Picton, P. (2000) *Neural Networks*, 2nd edn, Basingstoke: Palgrave.

Richards, P. (1985) *Indigenous Agricultural Revolution: Ecology and food production in West Africa*, London: Hutchinson.

—— (1986) *Coping with Hunger: Hazard and experiment in a West African rice farming system*, London: Allen and Unwin.

—— (2015) 'A matter of grave concern? Charles Jedrej's work on Mende sodalities, and the Ebola crisis', *Critical African Studies*, 13 November, doi: 10.1080/21681392.2016.1099021.

Richards, P., M. De Bruin-Hoekzema, S. G. Hughes, C. Kudadjie-Freeman, S. S. Offei, S. Kwame, C. Paul and A. Zannou (2009) 'Seed systems for African food security: linking molecular genetic analysis and cultural knowledge in West Africa', *International Journal of Technology Management*, 45: 196–214.

Richards, P., J. Amara, M. C. Ferme, P. Kamara, E. Mokuwa, I. A. Sheriff, R. Suluku and M. Voors (2015) 'Social pathways for Ebola Virus Disease in rural Sierra Leone, and some implications for containment', *PLOS Neglected Tropical Diseases*, 17 April, doi: 10.1371/journal.pntd.0003567.

Scarpino, S., A. Iamarino et al. (2014) 'Epidemiological and viral genomic sequence analysis of the 2014 Ebola outbreak reveals clustered transmission', *Clinical Infectious Diseases*, 60(7): 1079–82, 18 December.

Schlanger, N. (ed.) (2006) *Marcel Mauss: Techniques, technology and civilisation*, New York/Oxford: Durkheim Press/Berghahn Books.

Sharma, A. et al. (2014) 'Evidence for a decrease in transmission of Ebola virus – Lofa County, Liberia, June 8–November 1, 2014', *Morbidity and Mortality Weekly Report*, Centers for Disease Control and Prevention, 21 November, 63(46): 1067–71.

Simmel, G. (1906) 'The sociology of secrecy and of the secret societies', *American Journal of Sociology*, 11: 441–98.

Stadler, T., D. Kühnert, D. A. Rasmussen and L. du Plessis (2014) 'Insights into the early epidemic spread of Ebola in Sierra Leone provided by Viral Sequence Data', *PLOS Currents Outbreaks*, 1, 6 October, doi: 10.1371/currents.outbreaks.02bc6d927ecee7bbd33532ec8ba6a25f.

Sterne, J. (2003) 'Bourdieu, technique and technology', *Cultural Studies*, 17(3/4): 367–89.

Tawney, R. H. (1977 [1926]) *Religion and the Rise of Capitalism*, Harmondsworth: Penguin.

Van der Niet, A. G. (2009) 'Bodies in action: the influence of culture on body movements and skills in football and mundane daily life in post conflict Sierra Leone', Thesis, Research Masters Degree in African Studies, Leiden University.

Weber, M. (1930) *The Protestant Ethic and the Spirit of Capitalism*, trans. T. Parsons, London and New York: Routledge.

Weitz, J. S. and J. Dushoff (2015) 'Modeling post-death transmission of Ebola: challenges for inference and opportunities for control, *Nature, Scientific Reports*, 5, article no. 8751, 4 March, doi: 10.1038/srep08751.

WHO (World Health Organization) (2014a) 'Key messages for social mobilization and community engagement in intense transmission areas', Geneva: WHO, www.WHO/EVD/Guidance/socMob/14.1.

—— (2014b) 'Protocol on safe and dignified burial', apps.who.int/iris/bitstream/10665/137379/1/WHO_EVD_GUIDANCE_Burials_14.2_eng.pdf?ua=1.

Zamoyski, A. (2001) *Rites of Peace: The fall of Napoleon and the Congress of Vienna*, London: HarperPress.

INDEX